PEDIATRICS, CHILD AND ADOLESCENT HEALTH

ADVANCES IN PRETERM
INFANT RESEARCH

PEDIATRICS, CHILD AND ADOLESCENT HEALTH

JOAV MERRICK - SERIES EDITOR

NATIONAL INSTITUTE OF CHILD HEALTH
AND HUMAN DEVELOPMENT,
MINISTRY OF SOCIAL AFFAIRS, JERUSALEM

Child and Adolescent Health Yearbook 2012
Joav Merrick (Editor)
2012. ISBN: 978-1-61942-788-4
(Hardcover)
2012. ISBN: 978-1-61942-789-1
(E-book)

Child Health and Human Development Yearbook 2011
Joav Merrick (Editor)
2012. ISBN: 978-1-61942-969-7
(Hardcover)
2012. ISBN: 978-1-61942-970-3
(E-book)

Child and Adolescent Health Yearbook 2011
Joav Merrick (Editor)
2012. ISBN: 978-1-61942-782-2
(Hardcover)
2012. ISBN: 978-1-61942-783-9
(E-book)

Tropical Pediatrics: A Public Health Concern of International Proportions
Richard R Roach, Donald E Greydanus, Dilip R Patel, Douglas N Homnick and Joav Merrick (Editors)
2012. ISBN: 978-1-61942-831-7
(Hardcover)
2012. ISBN: 978-1-61942-840-9 (E-book)

Child Health and Human Development Yearbook 2012
Joav Merrick (Editor)
2012. ISBN: 978-1-61942-978-9
(Hardcover)
2012. ISBN: 978-1-61942-979-6
(E-book)

Developmental Issues in Chinese Adolescents
Daniel TL Shek, Rachel CF Sun and Joav Merrick (Editors)
2012. ISBN: 978-1-62081-262-4
(Hardcover)
2012. ISBN: 978-1-62081-270-9
(E-book)

Positive Youth Development:
Theory, Research and
Application
*Daniel TL Shek, Rachel CF Sun
and Joav Merrick (Editors)*
2012. ISBN: 978-1-62081-305-8
(Hardcover)
2012. ISBN: 978-1-62081-347-8
(E-book)

Understanding Autism Spectrum
Disorder: Current Research
Aspects
*Ditza A Zachor and Joav Merrick
(Editors)*
2012. ISBN: 978-1-62081-353-9
(Hardcover)
2012. ISBN: 978-1-62081-390-4
(E-book)

Positive Youth Development: A
New School Curriculum to Tackle
Adolescent Developmental Issues
*Hing Keung Ma, Daniel TL Shek
and Joav Merrick (Editors)*
2012. ISBN: 978-1-62081-384-3
(Hardcover)
2012. ISBN: 978-1-62081-385-0
(E-book)

Transition from Pediatric
to Adult Medical Care
*David Wood, John G. Reiss,
Maria E. Ferris, Linda R. Edwards
and Joav Merrick (Editors)*
2012. ISBN: 978-1-62081-409-3
(Hardcover)
2012. ISBN: 978-1-62081-412-3
(E-book)

Chinese Adolescent Development:
Economic Disadvantages, Parents
and Intrapersonal Development
*Daniel TL Shek, Rachel CF Sun
and Joav Merrick (Editors)*
2013. ISBN: 978-1-62618-622-4
(Hardcover)
2013. ISBN: 978-1-62618-694-1
(E-book)

University and College Students:
Health and Development Issues
for the Leaders of Tomorrow
*Daniel TL Shek, Rachel CF Sun
and Joav Merrick (Editors)*
2013. ISBN: 978-1-62618-586-9
(Hardcover)
2013. ISBN: 978-1-62618-612-5
(E-book)

Adolescence and Behavior Issues
in a Chinese Context
*Daniel TL Shek, Rachel CF Sun,
and Joav Merrick (Editors)*
2013. ISBN: 978-1-62618-614-9
(Hardcover)
2013. ISBN: 978-1-62618-692-7
(E-book)

Advances in Preterm Infant
Research
*Jing Sun, Nicholas Buys
and Joav Merrick*
2013. ISBN: 978-1-62618-696-5
(Hardcover)
2013. ISBN: 978-1-62618-775-7
(E-book)

PEDIATRICS, CHILD AND ADOLESCENT HEALTH

ADVANCES IN PRETERM INFANT RESEARCH

JING SUN
NICHOLAS BUYS
AND
JOAV MERRICK

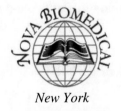

New York

Library of Congress Cataloging-in-Publication Data

ISBN: 978-1-692618-696-5

Library of Congress Control Number: 2013937384

Published by Nova Science Publishers, Inc. † New York

Contents

Preface

This book is a collection of a series of articles based on an Australian study that investigated executive function (EF) and sustained attention (SA) in preterm and full-term infants at eight months after expected date of delivery and at 10-11 months chronological age. Executive function and sustained attention emerge in infancy and continues to develop throughout childhood. Executive function and sustained attention is believed to underlie some learning problems in children at school age. Although numerous studies have reported that the overall development of preterm infants is comparable to that of full-term infants at the same corrected age, it is unclear to what extent the development of specific cognitive abilities is affected by prematurity and/or other factors such as medical complications. As preterm infants have a high rate of learning difficulties and attentional problems, it is possible that factors associated with prematurity specifically affect the development of some regions of the brain associated with the regulation of executive function and sustained attention.

Introduction

Senior lecturer Jing Sun, PhD[1], Professor Nicholas Buys, BA(Hons), MSc, PhD[2] and Professor Joav Merrick, MD, MMedSci, DMSc[3]

[1]School of Public Health, Griffith University and Griffith Health Institute, Griffith University, Gold Coast Campus, Meadowbrook, Australia
[2]School of Human Services and Social Work and Griffith Health Institute, Griffith University, Parkland, Gold Coast, Australia
[3]Medical Director, Health Services, Division for Intellectual and Developmental Disabilities, Ministry of Social Affairs and Social Services

This book is the experience from an Australian study that investigated executive function (EF) and sustained attention (SA) in preterm and full-term infants at 8 months after expected date of delivery and at 10-11 months chronological age. Executive function and sustained attention emerge in infancy and continues to develop throughout childhood. Executive function and sustained attention is believed to underlie some learning problems in children at school age. Although numerous studies have reported that the overall development of preterm infants is comparable to that of full-term infants at the same corrected age, it is unclear to what extent the development of specific cognitive abilities is affected by prematurity and/or other factors such as medical complications. As preterm infants have a high rate of learning difficulties and attentional problems, it is possible that factors associated with prematurity specifically affect the development of some regions of the brain associated with the regulation of executive function and sustained attention.

Thirty-seven preterm infants without identified disabilities, and 74 due date and gender matched healthy full-term infants, participated in the study. The preterm infants were all less than 32 weeks gestation and less than 1500 grams birthweight. The findings of the study showed that preterm infants performed significantly more poorly than full-term infants at both 8 months after the expected date of delivery and 10-11 months chronological age on all measures of executive function and sustained attention. However the difference between preterm and full-term infants at 8 months after expected date of delivery was much less than at 10-11 months chronological age. The results suggested that the effects of maturation are greater than the effects of exposure to extrauterine environmental stimuli on the development of executive function and sustained attention.

The four components of executive function (i.e., working memory, inhibition to prepotent response, inhibition to distration, and planning) did not correlate with each other when only infants with Bayley psychomotor ability scores greater than 85 were included, suggesting that the components of executive function may be discrete abilities which are governed by different parts of the prefrontal cortex. Sustained attention correlated with planning, supporting the suggestion that it may be a cognitive dimension which overlaps with executive function, depending upon the task requirement. Neither executive function nor sustained attention correlated with the Bayley mental ability and Bayley psychomotor ability scores when infants with scores of < 85 were excluded. This suggests that executive function and sustained attention measures are independent of general development.

In chapter 1 the background of the research program is presented. It focuses on the discussion in the literature in relation to the executive function deficits and neuropsychological development in preterm born children. Chapters 2, 3, 4, 5 present a comparison of executive function and sustained attention between preterm and full-term infants. This includes the working memory of preterm infants (chapter 2), the inhibitions (chapter 3), planning in preterm infants (chapter 4), and sustained attention in chapter 5.

The relationship between general development and executive function is discussed in chapter 6, which focuses on the general development measure and its relationship with executive function in this study, and chapter 7 then concludes the book chapters by discussing the limitation of the current research and its implications for further research and early intervention with preterm infants.

Chapter I

A review on early executive function deficit in preterm children and its association with neurodevelopmental disorders in childhood

Abstract

The purpose is to examine the association of deficits of executive function (EF) and neurodevelopmental disorders in preterm children, and the potential of assessing executive function in infants as means of early identification. Executive function refers to a collection of related but somewhat discrete abilities, the main ones being working memory, inhibition, and planning. There is a general consensus that EF governs goal-directed behaviour that requires holding those plans or programs on-line until executed, inhibiting irrelevant action, and planning a sequence of actions. Executive function plays an essential role in cognitive development and vital to individual social and intellectual success. Most researchers believe in the coordination and integrate cognitive-perceptual processes in relation to time and space, thus regulating higher-order cognitive processes such as problem solving, reasoning, logical, flexible thinking and decision making. The importance of the maturation of the frontal lobe, particularly the prefrontal cortex, to the development of EF in childhood has been emphasised. Therefore any abnormal development in the prefrontal lobes of infants and children could be expected to result in significant deficits in cognitive functioning. As this is a late-maturing part of the brain, various neurodevelopmental disorders, such as autism spectrum disorders, attention deficit hyperactivity disorder, language disorders and schizophrenia, as well as acquired disorders of the right brain (and traumatic brain injury) impair EF, the prefrontal cortex may be particularly susceptible to delayed development in these populations. The deficits of EF in infants are persistent into childhood and related to neurodevelopmental disorders in childhood and adolescence.

Introduction

There is increasing incidence of preterm delivery and the survival rate of preterm newborns is rising due to the advanced assisted reproductive technology and the improvement of technology in obstetrics and in neonatology. The survival rate in preterm birth is increasing with progressive increasing gestational ages (1) due to the improvement of neonatal intensive care. The survival rate of infants born at 25–25 weeks of gestation was 88 to 100% in 2010 (2) compared to 36-47% in1994 (3). In preterm newborns, prenatal, perinatal, and postnatal factors can give rise to adverse neurological outcomes through complex causal pathways (4). The main factors are brain injury (i.e. White Matter Damage, intraventricular hemorrhage, periventricular hemorrhage, and cortical and deep gray matter damage), and subsequent adverse clinical outcomes and increased incidence of disabilities increase with decreasing gestational age (5). As a significant proportion of brain growth, development, and networking occur approximately during the last 6 weeks of gestation (6), any injury or medical complications in the brain during this time can lead to adverse neurodevelopmental outcomes. The spectrum of neuro-developmental disorders in preterm children is wide and is represented by cerebral palsy (CP), developmental coordination disorder (DCD), neurosensorial impairment, including peripheral and/or central hearing and visual impairments, cognitive impairment, learning disabilities, and psychiatric disorders (i.e. attention deficit hyperactivity disorder, conduct problems, and emotional symptoms (7). These disorders have been found to be related to executive function deficits (4,8).

Executive function refers to a collection of high order cognitive abilities, the main ones being working memory, inhibition, planning, flexibility, and shift attention (9,10). There is a general consensus that EF governs goal-directed behaviour that requires holding those plans or programs on-line until executed, inhibiting irrelevant action, planning a sequence of actions, attention to distraction, being able to flexibly adjust to changed circumstances or new information (9). Executive function plays an essential role in cognitive development and is vital to the individual's social and intellectual success. It is thought by most researchers to coordinate and integrate cognitive-perceptual processes in relation to time and space, thus regulating higher-order executive functions such as problem solving, reasoning, logical and flexible thinking, and decision making.

The importance of the maturation of the frontal lobe, and in particular the prefrontal cortex, to the development of EF in childhood has been emphasised by several researchers. Given the important role of EF in cognitive development, any abnormal development in the prefrontal lobes of infants and children could be expected to result in significant deficits in cognitive functioning (11,12). As this is a late-maturing part of the brain, various neurodevelopmental disorders, such as autism spectrum disorders, attention deficit hyperactivity disorder, developmental language disorders, and schizophrenia, as well as acquired disorders of the right brain (and traumatic brain injury) impair EF, the prefrontal cortex may be particularly susceptible to delayed development in these populations. The current review aims to:

1. Examine the relationship between preterm birth and the development of prefrontal cortex and EF deficits;
2. Describe EF deficits in infants that persist into childhood and are related to neurodevelopmental disorders in childhood;
3. Explore possible assessment approaches to infant executive function through early identification of EF deficits.

The development of the prefrontal cortex in infants

Early birth has an influence on brain development and timing of neurobiological processes (13). These processes include neuronal migration and differentiation, axon and dendrite sprouting, synapse formation, myelination, programmed cell death, and the persistence of transient structures (i.e., the subplate). Compared to animals, the central nervous system of humans is late to reach full maturity when measured in terms of the number and volume of cells and the size and number of the dendritic spines of its neurons (14). Brain development begins early and advances quickly during the prenatal months, starting within the first month after conception, when the brain and spinal cord begin to take shape within the embryo. By the sixth prenatal month, nearly all of the billions of neurons (nerve cells) that populate the mature brain have been created, with new neurons generated at an average rate of more than 250,000 per minute. Neuronal proliferation and migration are completed well before birth. The outgrowth of axons and dendrites, myelination, synapse formation, and production of neurotransmitters also begins before birth and continues during the first 2 years of life. Once formed neurons quickly migrate to different parts of the brain and become differentiated to assume specialised roles, so that at birth, the majority of neurons are appropriately located within the immature brain. Neurones form connections (synapses) with other neurons enabling them to communicate and store information. These synapses continue to form throughout childhood. Axon outgrowth is followed by myelination. Some tracts are myelinated very early (i.e., antenatally), such as the vestibular tracts and some of the motor tracts; others are myelinated much later (e.g., the optical nerves, the auditory system, the cerebellar tracts, and prefrontal cortex).

The timetable for brain development varies by region, and continues throughout life. Sensory regions, which govern sight, touch, hearing, and other sensations, undergo their most rapid growth early in life, while the brain areas, such as the prefrontal cortex which guide higher forms of cognitive thinking and reasoning, continue to experience blooming and pruning of brain connections into early adolescence (14). The prefrontal cortex is one of the last regions of the central nervous system to undergo full myelination, and developmental changes originating from frontal lobe development are evident in several periods of life (14). The most active periods of development of the prefrontal cortex appear to be in the first 2 years of life, then between 7 and 9 years, and finally in adolescence.

The development of the frontal lobe in infants deserves particular mention because during this period remarkable and rapid changes occur in both the neural physiology and the behaviour of the human being. For the frontal cortex, the period of maximum synaptic excess appears to be in the second half of the first year (15), after which there occurs a protracted period of decline in synaptic density through selective elimination of little used pathways. Studies of human brain activity using PET documented developmental changes in rates of glucose metabolism (16). These changes are characterised by a rise in metabolism in the frontal region at approximately 6-8 months of age, followed by a prolonged period of decline in rates of metabolism which parallels the decline in synaptic density (16). Thus, it seems that the significant and rapid changes related to anatomy and function of the frontal lobe occur in the second half of the first year after birth and continue more slowly after this early period.

There is ample evidence that EF also develops dramatically during the second half of the first year of life. For example, infants can hold information in mind for increasing periods of time and use this information to direct and regulate their responses. They begin to inhibit prepotent responses (17) and become planful, demonstrating the ability to carry out relatively complex sequences of novel behavior (17). Behaviours of this type have been shown in numerous studies to be related to various areas of the prefrontal cortex.

The relation between executive function and the prefrontal cortex in human infants

Diamond and her colleagues (18) were the first to combine developmental psychology approaches with those of neuropsychology and comparative psychology to assess EF in both animal and human infants using the classic DR task and the A*B* task. The DR task procedure was originally used almost exclusively with animals. It requires the subject to watch the experimenter hide an attractive object in one of two identical wells. After a brief delay (the duration of which can be varied) the subject is allowed to search for the object. This sequence is repeated on subsequent trials with the hiding location changed randomly between the two wells.

The standard A*B* task was originally described by Piaget (19) to measure the changes in the concept of object permanence in human infants. In Piaget's A*B* task, an infant sits before two identical hiding places, often referred to as occluders (e.g., two identical cloth covers or two identical lids) that are separated by a small distance. While the infant watches, a desired object is hidden in one location (A). After a delay, the infant is allowed to reach and search for the object. This hiding and search at location A is repeated. Then while the infant watches, the object is hidden at the second location (B). After the delay, the infant is allowed to reach and search for the object. Infants frequently make the error of searching again at location A, committing what is known as the classic A*B* error. The A*B* task has undergone some minor modifications over time so that it allows the effects of time delay on search behaviour in human infants to be examined (10). It has many similarities to the DR task but varies in terms of the rules governing when the hiding place is changed.

The performance on DR tasks is believed to be governed by the prefrontal cortex (21). Studies using the DR task with infant monkeys have shown that they are able to retrieve a hidden object. However, when their frontal lobe is lesioned they are no longer able to carry out this task successfully (22). Diamond, Zola-Morgan, and Squire (23) found there were similarities in the pattern of the performance on the DR and A*B* tasks in primates. Infant monkeys with lesions of the dorsolateral prefrontal cortex showed errors at delays of 2 s and random or deteriorated performance at delays of 10 s on the A*B* task, despite their extensive preoperative training and their excellent performance with delays of 12 s before surgery. No recovery of performance occurred in the weeks following surgery (23). In addition, monkeys with dorsolateral prefrontal cortex lesions had poorer performance on the A*B* task than monkeys with lesions to the hippocampus formation.

Given the evidence of a link between the DR task and the prefrontal cortex, and the similarities in performance on the DR and A*B* task in primates, Diamond (24) suggested that the performance of human infants on the A*B* task may also be governed by the prefrontal cortex. If this is the case, the prefrontal cortex (which had been thought to be dormant in infancy) must be operating if only at a rudimentary level. Further support for this hypothesis came from a study by Diamond and Doar (18), which showed that human infants and infant monkeys display a similar progressive increase in successful performance on A*B* and DR tasks although at somewhat different ages. Human infants begin to carry out these tasks successfully at 7 ½ –8 months of age, and show improvement in performance up to about 12 months of age; whilst infant monkeys begin to carry out the task at 1½ months, and show improvement up to 2½ months. It was suggested that these advances may be due at least to maturational changes in the dorsolateral prefrontal cortex and proliferation of callosal connections between the supplementary motor areas of the left and right hemisphere (22). Although the dorsolateral prefrontal cortex is not fully mature in human infants of 7-12 months, it appears that at this age it has reached a level of maturity where it can support some critical cognitive functions.

The measurement of frontal scalp-recorded electroencephalograms (EEG) has given more credence to the relationship between the frontal cortex and performance on the A*B* task in human infants. Bell and Fox (25) were able to demonstrate a relationship between individual differences in frontal-brain electrical activity, as shown in EEG recordings and performance on the A*B* task. Infants at eight months of age who succeeded on the A*B* task exhibited greater power values in the frontal EEG during baseline recordings than infants who were unable to do the task (25,26). Additional evidence for the importance of prefrontal cortex maturation for the development of EF abilities has come from studies of children with phenylketonuria (27). Even when treated, this genetically transmitted error of metabolism can have the specific consequence of reducing the levels of the neurotransmitter dopamine in the dorsolateral prefrontal cortex. This results in impaired performance on tasks thought to measure EF, such as the A*B* task. Thus both electrophysiological and behavioural data provide support for the relation between the development of the prefrontal cortex and the emergence of EF in the first year of life.

Preterm birth and prefrontal cortex deficits

As the prefrontal cortex is one of the last regions of the central nervous system to undergo full myelination and is consequently one of the most immature parts of the brain at birth, any hazardous events may have a particularly detrimental effect on its development. The foundation for later brain development is established in the early years, however, the rapid pace and broad scope of early brain growth means that the immature brain is a vulnerable organ. Fetuses of 22 to 32 weeks gestation are now viable if cared for in intensive care nurseries. The brain at this point in development is a thin shell of tissue surrounding the cerebral ventricles. Neuroimaging studies using MRI technique have shown a significant association between brain volumes and gestational age at birth suggesting that brain development is associated with the degree of fetal immaturity when the transition from intrauterine to extrauterine life occurs. This transition may profoundly disrupt fetal brain development in preterm infants. However, brain development in preterm infants is imperiled by not only by exposure to stressful physiological changes, which it is ill prepared for, in the transition from intrauterine to extrauterine environment, but also by medical complications, and maternal distress during and after birth.

During this important maturation process in the first year of life, any damage or disturbance to the development of the prefrontal cortex due to disease, trauma, or conditions associated with perinatal risk factors (i.e., extremely low birthweight, shorter gestation age, and medical complications) may therefore lead to executive dysfunction. Diamond and Goldman-Rakic (28) used animal models to examine whether lesions of the dorsolateral prefrontal cortex would have the same effect on infant monkeys as on adult monkeys. Two of the infant rhesus monkeys were tested longitudinally on the A*B* and the DR tasks. They received bilateral lesions of the dorsolateral prefrontal cortex at 5½ months. They were then tested on the A*B* task at 6 months. The findings showed that the infant monkeys that had the prefrontal lesions displayed poorer performance on the A*B* task than their age mates who did not have the prefrontal lesions. The lesions produced the same effect in infant monkeys as they did in adult monkeys with prefrontal lesions: they all reached incorrectly when the delay increased to 2-5 s after the toy changed to the new hiding position.

The prefrontal cortex of infants who are born preterm is even more immature and prone to damage from the multitude of adverse medical complications to which these frail infants may be exposed. Lesions or atypical development of the prefrontal cortex occurring as a consequence of these hazardous events may have a detrimental effect on the development of EF which may have long-term consequences in terms of learning difficulties at school age. Indeed it has been found that children born preterm are at an increased risk for neurodevelopmental disorders when they reach school age and it has been suggested that this may be due to early abnormality in the development of the prefrontal cortex and consequently of executive dysfunction (29).

A range of different brain injuries are associated with premature birth that could affect neuropsychological outcomes. Large fluctuations in blood pressure in immature vessels can lead to hemorrhage in the germinal matrix. This may result in intraventricular hemorrhage and ventricular dilatation. Back pressure venous infarction may then occur, leading to a range of focal white and grey matter injuries, frequently associated with the later development of cerebral palsy. Fluctuations in brain perfusion may also lead to "watershed injury" in the periventricular white matter (periventricular leukcomalacia [PVL]) (30), which too may be associated with cerebral palsy in a proportion of cases. PVL is seen in 1% to 3% of preterm infants (31,32). Mortality in preterm infants with PVL ranges between 30% and 60% (32). Although mortality has decreased during the last years, PVL is still considered a disastrous lesion and is associated with adverse neurodevelopmental outcomes with motor, perceptual, and cognitive deficits (33,34). Most preterm infants with peri ventricular haemor.Most preterm infants with periventricular hemorrhage.

Executive function in preterm infants

Damage to the prefrontal lobe due to trauma and disease in infancy may have lifelong effects on EF abilities, and may cause neurodevelopmental disorders during school years (4,35,36). In comparison with adults, childhood frontal lobe lesions produce a more pervasive impairment, interfering with the acquisition of age-appropriate EF skills. Most studies on the relationship between EF development and frontal lobe damage in children are based on older children)(11,37). However, a case study by Anderson, Damasio, Tranel, and Damasio (38) reported that an infant who had right frontal region damage at 3 months showed severe learning difficulties and behavioural problems at school, and failure in career development in adulthood despite average intelligence (as measured by traditional intelligence tests at school age and during adulthood). The study found that the impairments largely reflected a failure to develop specific EFs, such as the ability to adapt to new situations, inhibit prepotent responses, and plan a sequence of actions to achieve a designated goal. These findings are consistent with the notion that early damage to prefrontal regions can lead to severe disruption of EF, while not significantly affecting many aspects tapped by standard intelligence tests. They also suggest that the prefrontal cortex may have limited neuronal plasticity which contributes to executive dysfunction if the damage occurs early. This may be due to disruption to the laying down of the neural architectures which are viewed as the foundation of cognitive development. A detailed examination of the relationship between prefrontal cortex development and the development of EF in a large sample of human infants has not been possible because of the relative lack of obvious prefrontal lesions in infants and the expense and lack of availability of neural imaging technology.

The development of EF as reflected in working memory, inhibition, and planning is age-related. Infants at seven to eight months of age start to display the ability to hold information in mind, inhibit prepotent and irrelevant responses, and execute and plan a course of action. These abilities continue to develop rapidly during childhood and adolescence. Any abnormality of the development of EF during this growth period may result in enduring neurodevelopment disorders. A number of investigators have proposed that neurodevelopmental disorders identified in preterm children are linked to impairments of one or more of the components of EF (4,8,39).

Deficits of working memory

Working memory, one of the major components of EF, is developing at age 8 to 12 months of age. Likewise in a study of children at 23 months and 66 months of age, the older children were found to have better performance on the delayed alternation task than the younger children (40) indicating continued improvement in working memory. Swanson (41) studied an even older age group (6 to 76 years of age) and found that performance on working memory tasks improved from 6 to 24 years of age, and then gradually started to decline at around age 35. This suggests that working memory continues to improve throughout childhood and into young adulthood (41,42).

Performance on achievement measures of both reading and mathematics has been found to be associated with measures of both verbal and non-verbal working memory ability (41). Preterm infants aged 8-10 month have been found have poorer performance than full term counterparts in working memory as measured by A*B* task (43). Similarly, preterm children with learning difficulties and low academic achievement at school age have been found to have visual-spatial working memory and verbal working memory deficits (44). For example, problem solving of mathematical word problems is a complex task that requires numerous cognitive operations such as comprehension, reasoning, and calculation. Prabhakaran, Bypma, and Gabrieli (45) suggested that multiple calculations with intermediate steps (e.g., 981 × 87) are dependent upon frontal lobe functioning. This may be due to an increase in working memory demands necessary for maintenance and manipulation of intermediate steps while problem solving. Verbal working memory is particularly important for the storage and rehearsal of speech-based verbal information and has been found to play a specialised role in reading comprehension (46). Impaired memory for digit span and non-word repetition, which measure verbal working memory, has been associated with learning difficulties in preterm children (44). The sense of past and future, afforded by working memory, gives the individual the capacity to understand the content in learning. However, preterm children with neurodevelopmental disorders have difficulty holding events in working memory (44)and consequently they are less able to formulate future plans than to respond to present events and less able to generate and select response options.

Deficits of inhibition

The ability to inhibit a prepotent response is also age-related, and like working memory, is first demonstrated at about 7-12 months of age (18), with improvements occurring between 18 and 30 months (47) in the primary school years (6-12 years) and again in young adults (18-29 years) (48). According to Barkley (49), deficient inhibition refers to impulsive acts or acting without thinking about the consequences. He described three components of inhibition, namely inhibition of a prepotent response, interruption of an ongoing response, and inhibition of interference from external stimuli. It has been found that preterm children with learning difficulties also frequently have attention deficits. In a population-based epidemiological study, it has been found that preterm children had attention deficits (50). Preterm children have been found consistently to have deficits in all three aspects of inhibition (7,51,52). This impairs the ability of children with learning difficulties or attention deficits to engage in other appropriate and more timely activities. Consequently, these children miss out opportunities to learn. Tasks assessing inhibition typically require an inappropriate response to be inhibited and irrelevant stimulus to be ignored. In a number of inhibition tasks such as the Go/No-Go task (53) and the Stroop Word-Color Test (54), and Walk not Walk task, preterm children showed poorer performance than typically developing children (55,56).

Deficits of planning

Sun and colleagues (17,43) found that planning ability similarly emerges in infants at 7-8 months of age, and Chen, Sanchez and Campbell (57) showed that children at 13 months of age were able to plan and execute the necessary course of action to solve age-appropriate problems and use flexibility in the choice of strategies to solve the problems. Bauer et al [58] reported that at 18 to 27 months of age children had developed the ability to represent the goal state of a problem and to plan, monitor, and execute a course of action necessary to achieve it.

The planning tasks used with children under two years of age typically require them to remove an obstacle to attain a goal. Older children are usually required to generate a path to a goal. For example, the Tower of Hanoi, which requires children to plan a course of action to reach the goal state, has been used with children from 3 years of age, with marked improvements in performance being observed from the ages of three to twelve, when adult levels of performance are achieved (42,59).

Performance on planning tasks has been found to correlate significantly with arithmetic computation and written composition test scores (60,61). Planning involves the delineation of steps or sequences, both cognitive and behavioural, that the individual will follow during the course of action (58,62). Problems with planning may manifest as difficulty sequencing information in temporal order, which may affect syntax of verbal expression and composition in writing, leading to low school achievement in these areas.

Planning also involves the application of systematic strategies rather than trial and error responses in reaching the goal (63). Strategies can be used to guide behaviour more efficiently and effectively. Such strategies are often critical to managing complex work or problem-solving tasks, particularly where subsets of strategy-guided behaviour must be organised into a larger hierarchy to accomplish tasks or goals.

Like patients with frontal lobe injuries who are often found to be deficient in task performances due to poor utilisation of strategies (64), preterm children with neurodevelopmental disorders have been found to be deficient in the formulation and application of strategies (65).

Tasks assessing planning typically require a sequence of steps to be planned, executed, monitored and revised in advance of action. The Tower of London and Tower of Hanoi tasks, which are classic tasks for the assessment of planning, require the planning of a series of moves, which are constrained by the rules of the task, in order to move from the start state to the required end state. Preterm children with learning difficulties have been found to have longer latencies (planning time) before commencing on Tower of London problems (66).

Early assessment of executive function

As early brain insult would have long-term implications for neurobehavioral outcome in preterm born infants, and the neurodevelopment disorders are related to the deficits of executive function, early identification executive function deficits in this population is crucial to inform early intervention and prevention practice.

Historically, the assessment of EF in infants was thought impossible. However, recent neuropsychological research has suggested that the AB task and infant planning tasks (17) provide avenues for research on working memory, inhibition of prepotent responses, inhibition of distraction, and planning, which are considered to be components of EF. Similar to the assessment of EF for adults and older children, the assessment of EF in infants also requires working memory, inhibition, and planning. It has been found that the AB task and planning tasks in infants require these components of EF (17,28,62,67).

A*B* tasks

In addition to being able to mentally represent the object, the following abilities are required for infants to carry out the A*B* task successfully: 1) memory of the object's hiding location; 2) inhibition of the prepotent response to the previously correct location; and 3) inhibition of interference from external stimuli (24). Hence completion of this task clearly requires components of EF and it could therefore be regarded as a suitable means of assessing EF in human infants.

Working memory for the location of a hidden object

Performance on A*B* tasks may reflect the emergence of working memory (24,68). The evidence that strongly supports this is Diamond's (20) finding that performance on the A*B* task deteriorated with increasing delay between the time when the object was hidden and the time when the infant was allowed to search. This suggests that the memory of the hidden object becomes progressively weaker when the delay increases. The maximum time delay for correct object location in the A*B* task has been found to be 2 s for 7-8 month olds, 5 s at 9 months, and 10 s at 12 months (22). At each age, if the delay is reduced by 2-3 seconds, infants will reach correctly whether the toy is hidden at the first retrieval position or changed to another location. If the delay is increased by 2-3 seconds, they err even on location A. At all ages, infants' performances improve if they are allowed to strain towards the correct location during the delay (18). It seems that finding a hidden object in position A mostly requires working memory, and increasing the delay time between hiding and retrieval increases the difficulty of the task for infants.

Inhibition of prepotent responses

Several researchers (69, 70) have suggested that a combination of working memory deficits and inability to inhibit repetition of a previously rewarded response causes A*B* errors. Diamond suggested that the A*B* task sets up a conflict between the ability to use working memory to guide behaviour and a conditioned behavioural tendency to repeat a rewarded response when the object has been hidden at location B. Success at location A strengthens the tendency to reach to it by reinforcing this place response, and/or establishing a mental set for this response. The more frequently this response is reinforced the stronger the response tendency becomes. Infants of 8-12 months make A*B* errors because they fail to resist the 'reinforced habit' to repeat the previously successful responses at location A. This is evident from the study in which transparent occluders A and B were used, and infants still made A*B* errors although less frequently than when the occluders were opaque (71). Thus the learned habit seems at times to be stronger than even the attraction of the object.

Reaching to a previously rewarded location (location A) requires only working memory, but reaching to a new location (location B) requires both working memory and inhibition of the incorrect prepotent response, making the task more difficult and therefore more prone to errors. It is suggested that as the strength of the prepotent response increases due to repeated reinforcement, the ability to inhibit it must also increase if a correct response is to be made to a new location (72).

Inhibiting distraction from external stimuli

Interference control, or resistance to distraction, is defined by Barkley as the ability to "inhibit responding to sources of interference while engaged in another task requiring self-control or while delaying a response" (49). Whether or not distracters disrupt task performance depends upon the strength of the distracter and the potency of the response likely to be elicited by it (49). In the A*B* task, when a delay time is imposed between hiding and retrieval, external stimuli, such as the cover which is used to hide the object, may act as a distracter which interferes with the performance of the task. Few studies have, however, examined infants' ability to inhibit attention to distracter stimuli.

In summary, the analysis of performance on the A*B* task shows the importance of EF in completing this task. There is agreement that the EF abilities required to successfully carry out the A*B* task are working memory and inhibition of the prepotent response and consequently most studies have focused on these factors (20.69). It seems that inhibition to distraction from external stimuli is also required to conduct the A*B* task and few studies have examined this aspect of inhibition.

Planning task

The majority of research on planning by infants is based on their ability to negotiate means-ends problems that require overcoming obstacles to reach observable goals. For example, Sun and colleagues (17, 43) used a 1-step planning task in which infants were presented with a desired toy that was just out of their reach on the far end of a cloth. In order to reach the goal (toy), the infants had to pull the cloth. Infants younger than six months of age showed behaviour that was neither intentional nor goal-directed. For example, they often ignored the goal object or appeared surprised when they eventually noticed it (62).

At 7 to 8 months infants were able to sequence the necessary steps to get the toy showing planned, goal-directed action. By 10 months, infants were found to be able to solve more complex problems involving a sequence of two subgoals. For example, a 2-step planning task used by Willatts and Rosie (73) required the infants to remove a barrier to gain access to a cloth, then pull the cloth to bring the toy within reach. Infants at 10 months had the capacity to conceptualise the goal of retrieving the toy and could achieve the sub-goals of removing the barrier and pulling the cloth to bring the toy within reach so that it could be grasped. At 12 months, they could extend and chain simple means-ends skills in a 3-step problem-solving task which required the removal of a barrier to gain access to a cloth, pulling the cloth to retrieve a string, then pulling the string to bring the toy within reach (74). Infants show steady improvements in their ability to order their actions and to make either reaching or crawling detours when faced with barriers, so that they show flexibility in sequencing their actions and are able to create longer chains of temporally sequenced actions in order to obtain a desired goal (75,76).

In a cross-sectional study, Chen et al (57) compared groups of infants at 10 and 13 months on a more complex planning task. The task which they used was somewhat different from that used by Willatts and Rosie (74). In this task, a barrier was put in front of two pieces of cloth, each of which had a string on it. A toy was attached to one string but not to the other. The infant needed to remove the barrier, pull the relevant cloth, and then pull the string to bring the toy within reach. The solution to the problem required choosing the correct subgoal, such as selecting the relevant cloth in order to retrieve the toy. As suggested by Willatts (77), the planning task is more difficult when the infant must initially choose between two subgoals which determine the achievement of later ones. For example, if the infant chooses the irrelevant cloth (i.e., the one with a string which is not attached to toy), then no further action will be possible and the problem will remain unsolved. However, if the correct subgoal (i.e., correct cloth) is selected, then the infant can proceed to the next subgoal and will solve the problem. The ability to order a preferred sequence of actions in anticipation of goal conflict necessarily involves planning, which includes mentally representing the effects of first attempting to achieve each subgoal, noticing the conflict of two identical subgoals (such as two cloths), and finding the solution in advance of any action and without feedback. Findings in the study by Chen et al (57) showed that infants at both 10 and 13 months used a more or less trial-and-error approach and did not show any planned and intentional actions for the first trial because they could not detect the critical subgoal conflict. However, the performance of the 13 month infant group improved after modelling a solution, suggesting they recognised and understood the conflict even though they failed to plan how to avoid it. Willatts further suggested that the acquisition of this complex means-end strategy starts to develop after 12 months and continues well beyond the period of infancy. Cognitive tasks involving means-end problem solving, which is clearly planned intentionally with a goal in mind, have enabled the planning components of EF to be examined in infants.

Because planning tasks involve a number of steps there are opportunities for distracters to intervene and disrupt performance. Whether or not this occurs is likely to depend upon the power of the distracter, the level of prepotency of the response elicited by the distracting object or event, and conflict between the sub-goal and the goal (49,62). In the 1-step planning task, Willatts (62)found that although 6 month-old infants initially fixated on the toy, they often looked away, fixated on the cloth, picked it up, and played with it. Thus the immediate or closest stimulus, that is the cloth, acted as a distracter which interfered with the performance of the planning task. However by 7 to 8 months, infants planned in advance and inhibited distractions in order to sequence the steps and achieve the goal, such as retrieval of the toy. Clearly, completion of a planning task requires not only planning but also inhibition of distraction from external stimuli.

Conclusion

In summary, EF develops rapidly in childhood, with the components of working memory, inhibition, and planning emerging in infancy and improving steadily in the second half of the first year of life. Developmental problems with EF have been shown to underlie neurodevelopmental disorders including learning difficulties and attention deficits in children, and these problems are particularly common in children born preterm. Early assessment of these problems is critical to successful interventions to promote normal development of EF. The use of A*B* and planning tasks that require components of working memory, inhibition and planning make early identification of EF deficits in this population possible, and can therefore inform early intervention and prevention practice.

References

[1] Blondel B, Macfarlane A, Gissler M, Breart G, Zeitlin J, Group PS. Preterm birth and multiple pregnancy in European countries participating in the PERISTAT project. BJORG 2006;113(528-535).

[2] Michikata K, Sameshima H, Sumiyoshi K, Kodama Y, Kaneko M, Ikenoue T. Developmental changes in catecholamine requirement, volume load and corticosteroid supplementation in premature infants born at 22 to 28 weeks of gestation. Early Hum Dev 2010;86:401-5.

[3] Ferrara TB, Hoekstra RE, Couser RJ, Gaziano EP, Calvin SE, Payne NR, et al. Survival and follow-up of infants born 23 to 26 weeks of gestational age: Effects of surfactant therapy. J Pediatr 1994;124:119-24.

[4] Arpino C, Compagnone E, Montanaro ML, Cacciatore D, Luca AD, Cerulli A, et al. Preterm birth and neurodevelopmental outcome: a review. Child Nerv Syst. 2010;26:1139-49.

[5] McQuillen PS, Sheldon RA, Shatz CJ, Ferriero DA. Selective vulnerability of subplate neurons after early neonatal hypoxia-ischemia. J Neurosci. 2003;23(8):3308-15.

[6] Adams-Chapman I. Neurodevelopmental outcome of the late preterm infant. Clin Perinat. 2006;33:947-64.

[7] Marlow N, Hennessy EM, Bracewell MA, Wolke D. Motor and executive function at 6 years of age after extremely preterm birth. Pediatrics. 2007;120(4):793-804.

[8] Mulder H, Pitchford NJ, Marlow N. Processing speed and working memory underlie academic attainment in very preterm children. Arch Disabl Child Fetal Neonatal. 2010;95:F267-F72.

[9] Huizinga M, Dolan CV, van der Molen MW. Age-related change in executive function: Developmental trends and a latent variable analysis. Neuropsychologia. 2006;44:2017-36.

[10] Miyake A, Friedman NP, Emerson MJ, Witzki AH, Howerter A. The unity and diversity of executive functions and their contributions to complex "Frontal Lobe" tasks: A latent variable analysis. Cognitive Psychology. 2000;41:49-100.

[11] Eslinger PJ, Biddle K, Pennington B, Page RB. Cognitive and behavioral development up to 4 years after early right frontal lobe lesion. Dev Neuropsychol. 1999;15(2):157-91.

[12] Aanoudse-Moens CSH, Weisglas-Kuperus N, van Goudoever JB, Oosterlaan J. Meta-Analysis of Neurobehavioral Outcomes in Very Preterm and/or Very Low Birth Weight Children. Pediatrics. 2009;124(2):717-28.

[13] Volpe JJ. Brain injury in premature infants: a complex amalgam of destructive and developmental disturbances. Lancet Neurol. 2009;8:110-24.

[14] Gogtay N, Giedd JN, Lusk L, Hayashi KM, Greenstein D, Vaituzis AC, et al. Dynamic mapping of human cortical development during childhood through early adulthood. PNAS. 2004;101: 8174-9.

[15] Huttenlocher PR. Synaptogenesis in human cerebral cortex. In: Dawson G, Fischer KW, editors. Human behavior and the developing brain. New York: The Guilford Press; 1994. p. 137-52.

[16] Chugani HT, Phelps ME. Imaging human brain development with positron emission tomography. J Nucl Med. 1990;32:23-5.

[17] Sun J, Mohay H, O'Callaghan M. Executive function in preterm and full-term infants. Early Hum Dev. 2009;85(4):225-30.

[18] Diamond A, Doar B. The performance of human infants on a measure of frontal cortex function, the delayed response task. Dev Psychobiol. 1989;22(3):271-94.

[19] Piaget J. The construction of reality in the child. New York: Basic Books; 1954.

[20] Diamond A. Development of the ability to use recall to guide action, as indicated by infants' performance on A*B*. Child Dev. 1985;56:868-83.

[21] Diamond A, Kirkham N, Amso D. Conditions under which young children can hold two rules in mind and inhibit a prepotent response. Dev Psychol. 2002;38(3):352-62.

[22] Diamond A. Neuropsychological insights into the meaning of object concept development. In: Johnson MH, editor. Brain development and cognition: A reader. Cambridge, MA: Blackwell; 1993. p. 208-47.

[23] Diamond A, Zola-Morgan S, Squire LR. Successful performance by monkeys with lesions of the hippocampal formation on A*B* and Object Retrieval, two tasks that mark developmental changes in human infants. Behav Neurosc. 1989;103(3):526-37.

[24] Diamond A. The development and neural bases of memory functions as indexed by the A*B* and delayed response tasks in human infants and infant monkeys. The development and neural bases of higher cognitive functions: Annals of the New York Academy of Sciences. New York: The New York Academy of Sciences; 1990. p. 394-433.

[25] Bell MA, Fox NA. The relations between frontal brain electrical activity and cognitive development during infancy. Child Dev. 1992;63:1142-63.

[26] Bell MA. Frontal lobe function during infancy: Implications for the development of cognition and attention. In: Richards JE, editor. Cognitive neuroscience of attention: A developmental perspective. Mahwah, NJ: Lawrence Erlbaum; 1998. p. 287-316.

[27] Diamond A, Prevor MB, Callender G, Druin DP. Prefrontal cortex cognitive deficits in children treated early and continuously for PKU. Monogr Soc Res Child Dev. 1997;62(4):1-205.

[28] Diamond A, Goldman-Rakic PS. Comparative development of human infants and infant rhesus monkeys of cognitive functions that depend on the prefrontal cortex. Neuropsychol Abstr. 1986;12:274.

[29] Lowe J, Duvall SW, MacLean PC, Caprihan A, Ohls R, Qualls C, et al. Comparison of structural magnetic resonance imaging and development in toddlers born very low birthweight and full term. J Child Neurol. 2011;26(5):586-92.

[30] Rennie JM. The immature brain. In: Rennie JM, editor. Neonatal cerebral ultrasound. Cambridge: Cambridge University Press; 1997. p. 124.

[31] Hamrick SEG, Miller SP, Leonard C, et al. Trends in severe brain injury and neurodevelopmental outcome in premature newborn infants: the role of cystic periventricular leukomalacia. J Pediatr. 2004;145(5):593-9.

[32] Roze E, Kerstjens JM, Ter Horst HJ, Maathuis CGB, Bos AF. Risk factors for adverse outcome in preterm infants with periventricular hemorrhagic infarction. . 2008;122(1). Pediatrics. 2008;122(1).

[33] Bassan H, Limperopoulos C, Visconti K, et al. Neurodevelopmental outcome in survivors of periventricular hemorrhagic infarction. Pediatrics Pediatrics. 2007;120(4):785-92.

[34] Brouwer A, Groenendaal F, van Haastert IL, Rademaker K, Hanlo P, de Vries L. Neurodevelopmental outcome of preterm infants with severe intraventricular hemorrhage and therapy for post-hemorrhagic ventricular dilatation. J Pediatr. 2008;152(5):648–54.

[35] Eslinger PJ, Grattan LM, Damasio H, Damasio AR. Developmental consequences of childhood frontal lobe damage. Arch Neurol. 1992;49:764-9.

[36] Scheibel RS, Levin HS. Frontal lobe dysfunction following closed head injury in children: Findings from neuropsychology and brain imaging. In: Krasnegor NA, Lyon GR, Goldman-Rakic PS, editors. Development of the prefrontal cortex: Evolution, neurobiology, and behavior. Baltimore: Paul H. Brookes; 1997. p. 241-63.

[37] Mateer CA, Williams D. Effects of frontal lobe injury in childhood. Dev Neuropsychol. 1991;7(2):359-76.

[38] Anderson SW, Damasio H, Tranel D, Damasio AR. Long-term sequelae of prefrontal cortex damage acquired in early childhood. Dev Neuropsychol. 2000;18(3):281-90.

[39] Mulder H, Pitchford NJ, Hagger MS, Marlow N. Development of Executive Function and Attention in Preterm Children: A Systematic Review. Dev Neuropsychol. 2009;34(4):393-421.

[40] Espy KA, Kaufmann PM, McDiarmid MD, Glisky ML. Executive functioning in preschool children: Performance on A-not-B and other delayed response format tasks. Brain Cogn. 1999;41:178-99.

[41] Swanson HL. What develops in working memory? A life span perspective. Dev Psychol. 1999;35(4):986-1000.

[42] Welsh MC, Pennington BF, Groisser DB. A normative-developmental study of executive function: A window on prefrontal function in children. Dev Neuropsychol. 1991;7(2):131-49.

[43] Sun J, Buys N. Prefrontal lobe functioning and its relationship to working memory in preterm infants. Int J Child Adolesc Health. 2011;4(1):13-7.

[44] Gathercole SE, Pickering SJ. Working memory deficits in children with low achievements in the national curriculum at 7 years of age. Br J Dev Psychol. 2000; 70:177-94.

[45] Prabhakaran V, Rypma B, Gabrieli JDE. Neural substrates of mathematical reasoning: A functional magnetic resonance imaging study of neocortical activation during performance of the necessary arithmetic operations tests. Neuropsychology. 2001;15(1):115-27.

[46] Nation K, Adams JW, Bowyer-Crane CA, Snowling MJ. Working memory deficits in poor comprehenders reflect underlying language impairments. J Exp Child Psychol. 1999;73:139-58.

[47] Vaughn BE, Kopp CB, Krakow JB. The emergence and consolidation of self-control from eighteen to thirty months of age: Normative trends and individual differences. Child Dev. 1984;55:990-1004.

[48] Williams BR, Ponesse JS, Schachar RJ, Logan GD, Tannock R. Development of inhibitory control across the life span. Dev Psychol. 1999;35(1):205-13.

[49] Barkley RA. Behavioral inhibition, sustained attention, and executive functions: Constructing a unifying theory of ADHD. Psychol Bull. 1997;121(1):65-94.

[50] Harvey JM, O'Callaghan MJ, Mohay H. Executive function of children with extremely low birthweight: A case control study. Dev Med Child Neurol. 1999;41:292-7.

[51] Bohm B, Katz-Salamon M, Smedler A, Lagercrantz H, Forssberg H. Developmental risks and protective factors for influencing cognitive outcome at 5 1/2 years of age in very-low-birthweight children. Dev Med Child Neurol. 2002;44:508-16.

[52] Katz KS, Dubowitz LM, Henderson S, Jongmans M, Kay GG, Nolte CA. Effect of cerebral lesions on continuous performance test responses of school age children born prematurely. J Pediatr Psychol. 1996;21(6):841-55.

[53] Schachar R, Mota VL, Logan GD, Tannock R, Klim P. Confirmation of an inhibitory control deficit in attention-deficit/hyperactivity disorder. J Abnorm Child Psychol. 2000;28(3):227-35.

[54] Pennington BF, Groisser D, Welsh MC. Contrasting cognitive deficits in attention deficit hyperactivity disorder versus reading disability. Dev Psychol. 1993;29(3):511-23.

[55] Atkinson J, Braddick O. Visual and visuocognitive development in children born very prematurely. Prog Brain Res. 2007;164:123-49.

[56] Bayless S, Stevenson J. Executive functions in school-age children born very prematurely. Early Hum Dev. 2007;84(4):247-54.

[57] Chen Z, Sanchez RP, Campbell T. From beyond to within their grasp: The rudiments of analogical problem solving in 10- and 13-month-olds. Dev Psychol. 1997;33(5):790-801.

[58] Bauer PJ, Schwade JA, Wewerka SS, Delaney K. Planning ahead: Goal-directed problem solving by 2-year-olds. Dev Psychol. 1999;35(5):1321-37.

[59] Passler MA, Isaac W, Hynd GW. Neuropsychological development of behavior attributed to frontal lobe functioning in children. Dev Neuropsychol. 1985;1(4):349-70.

[60] Hooper SR, Swartz CW, Wakely MB, de Kruif REL, Montgomery JW. Executive functions in elementary school children with and without problems in written expression. J Learn Disabil. 2002;35(1):57-68.

[61] Snow JH. Developmental patterns and use of the Wisconsin Card Sorting Test for children and adolescents with learning disabilities. Child Neuropsycho. 1998;4(2):89-97.

[62] Willatts P. Development of means-end behavior in young infants: Pulling a support to retrieve a distant object. Dev Psychol. 1999;35(3):651-67.

[63] Scholnick EK, Friedman SL. Planning in context: Developmental and situational considerations. Int J Behav Dev. 1993;16(2):145-67.

[64] Stuss DT, Eskes GA, Foster JK. Experimental neuropsychological studies of frontal lobe functions. In: Boller F, Spinnler H, Hendler JA, editors. Handbook of neuropsychology. Amsterdam: Elsevier; 1994. p. 149-85.

[65] Keeler ML, Swanson HL. Does strategy knowledge influence working memory in children with mathematical disabilities? J Learn Disabil. 2001;34(5):418-34.

[66] Luciana M, Lindeke L, Georgieff M, Mills M, Nelson CA. Neurobehavioral evidence for working-memory deficits in school-aged children with histories of prematurity. Dev Med Child Neurol. 1999;41:521-33.

[67] Diamond A. Frontal lobe involvement in cognitive changes during the first year of life. In: Gibson KR, Peterson AC, editors. Brain maturation and cognitive development: Comparative and cross-cultural perspectives Foundations of human behavior. New York: Aldine De Gruyter; 1991. p. 127-80.

[68] Gilmore RO, Johnson MH. Working memory in infancy: Six-month-olds' performance on two versions of the oculomotor delayed response task. J Exp Child Psychol. 1995;59:397-418.

[69] Diamond A. Abilities and neural mechanisms underlying A*B* performance. Child Dev. 1988;59:523-7.

[70] McCall DD, Clifton RK. Infants' means-end search for hidden objects in the absence of visual feedback. Infant Behav Dev. 1999;22:179-95.

[71] Butterworth G. Object disappearance and error in Piaget's stage IV task. J Exp Child Psychol. 1977;23: 391-401.

[72] Diamond A, Werker JF, Lalonde C. Toward understanding commonalities in the development of object search, detour navigation, categorization, and speech perception. In: Dawson G, Fischer KW, editors. Human behavior and the developing brain. New York: The Guilford Press; 1994. p. 380-426.

[73] Willatts P, Rosie K. Thinking ahead: Development of means-end planning in young infants. Infant Behav Dev. 1992;15:769.

[74] Willatts P, Rosie K, eds. Planning by 12-month-old infants. Annual Conference of the Society for Research in Child Development; 1989 April; Kansas City, MO.

[75] Lockman JJ, Pick HL. Problems of scale in spatial development. In: Sophian C, editor. Origins of cognitive skills. Hillsdale, NJ: Lawrence Erlbaum, 1984:3-26.

[76] McKenzie BE, Bigelow E. Detour behavior in young human infants. Br J Dev Psychol 1986;4:139-48.

[77] Willatts P, ed. Development of means-end planning in the second year of life. International Conference on Infant Studies; 1998 April; Atlanta, GA.

Chapter II

Inhibition and prefrontal lobe functioning in preterm and full-term infants

Abstract

This chapter examines inhibition in preterm at eight months after expected date of delivery (when preterm infants were actually 10-11 months chronological age) and full-term infants at eight months. Inhibition emerges in infancy and continues to develop throughout childhood. Inhibition is believed to underlie some behavioral and learning problems in children at school age. Thirty-seven preterm infants without identified disabilities, and 74 due date and gender matched healthy full-term infants, participated in the present study. The preterm infants were all less than 32 weeks gestation and less than 1,500 grams birthweight. All infants were therefore assessed on inhibition to prepotent response and inhibitioni to distraction of external stimuli tasks at 8 months after the expected date of delivery.

The findings of the study showed that preterm infants performed significantly more poorly than full-term infants at both eight months corrected age and 10-11 month chronological age on measures of in inhibition to prepotent response and inhibitioni to distraction of external stimuli tasks.

Medical risk, lower birthweight and lower gestation age were found significantly affect the performance on inhibition tasks. The results of this study suggests that the deficits of inhibition in preterm infants may be associated with lower birthweight, shorter gestatation and medical complications.

Introduction

Inhibition involving inhibiting prepotent responses and resisting distraction or disruption by competing events, and flexibility of thinking reflects cognitive perspective (1,2). Barkley (2) conceptualised inhibition as three interrelated abilities:

- *The ability to inhibit a prepotent response from occurring.* A prepotent response is a response which is established through reinforcement and is resistant to the changing circumstance. For example, in the situation where a choice must be made between two locations where a reward may be hidden, the prepotent response is established through reinforcement of one location (e.g., location A). When the reward is moved to a different location the subject is likely reaching back to the previously successful location. This is called an inability to inhibit a prepotent response. Prepotent responses may be elicited not only by external stimuli, but also by conditioned stimuli from the internal environment (i.e., thoughts, and emotions). Without the capacity to inhibit prepotent responses, new goals cannot be achieved and new learning will not take place.
- *The capacity to interrupt an ongoing sequence of behaviour.* If the feedback from a series of responses indicates the ongoing behaviours are erroneous or ineffective, then this sequence of behaviour must be interrupted. Thus the individual must exhibit flexibility that allows ongoing behaviour to be altered quickly in response to the changing situation. This requires a degree of self-monitoring and an awareness of immediate past responses and their outcomes.
- *Interference control, the ability to inhibit responding to irrelevant interference or distraction while engaging in a task.* Failure to do this leads to neglect of the relevant stimuli and increased attention to extraneous background stimuli. Thus distractibility, which is often a characteristic of children with attention deficit disorders, may be caused by inefficient response inhibition (2). The cognitive inhibition is different from social inhibition in studies of shy and socially inhibited children, in which the term "inhibition" refers to clinging, quiet, timid, shy and withdrawn behaviour (3-5).

Difficulty with inhibition of a prepotent response: Patients with frontal lobe damage also frequently fail to inhibit or suppress inappropriate or untimely actions which interfere with goal-directed behaviour, because their attention is vulnerable to interference from both external stimuli and internal representations or prepotent responses. As Fuster (6) expressed it, interference can come from sensory stimuli that appear in the context of the behavioural structure and that, if not suppressed, can lead the behaviour away from its goal. The interference can also be seen in the form of internal tendencies, whether inborn or the product of learning. For example, it may be interference from instinctual impulses that, under certain conditions, prevail over current behaviour and disrupt it. Or, alternatively, the interference may come from well-established memories or patterns of behaviour that are appropriate in other circumstances but are an impediment to current behaviour and the achievement of the goal (6). Failure to inhibit a prepotent response is responsible for poor performance on the Wisconsin Card Sorting Test (WCST), in which the subject must keep in mind the criteria for sorting a set of visual figures and be prepared to shift criteria when the sorting criteria change (7,8).

Difficulty in inhibiting distraction: Patients who have frontal lobe damage may be abnormally attracted by irrelevant stimuli, and be unable to resist the interference from stimuli that would normally be suppressed or ignored by adults who do not have frontal lobe damage (9,10). Thus, relevant stimuli appear to be neglected while attention to background or irrelevant stimuli isincreased. This failure to suppress extraneous information is reminiscent of the disorder of interference control that animals which have orbital prefrontal lesions exhibit in structured tasks (11-13). It implies disruption to an inhibitory control mechanism which would normally allow attention to be focused on stimuli which are germane to the task.

The development of the prefrontal cortex in infants

Compared to animals, the central nervous system of humans is late to reach full maturity when measured in terms of the number and volume of cells and the size and number of the dendritic spines of its neurons (14,15). Brain development begins early and advances quickly during the prenatal months starting within the first month after conception, when the brain and spinal cord begin to take shape within the embryo. By the sixth prenatal month, nearly all of the billions of neurons (nerve cells) that populate the mature brain have been created, with new neurons generated at an average rate of more than 250,000 per minute. Neuronal proliferation and migration are completed well before birth. The outgrowth of axons and dendrites, myelination, synapse formation, and production of neuro-transmitters also begins before birth and continues during the first two years of life. Once formed neurons quickly migrate to different parts of the brain and become differentiated to assume specialised roles, so that at birth, the majority of neurons are appropriately located within the immature brain. Neurones form connections (synapses) with other neurons enabling them to communicate and store information. These synapses continue to form throughout childhood. Axon outgrowth is followed by myelination. Some tracts are myelinated very early (i.e., antenatally), such as the vestibular tracts and some of the motor tracts; others are myelinated much later (e.g., the optical nerves, the auditory system, the cerebellar tracts, and prefrontal cortex).

The prefrontal cortex of infants who are born preterm is even more immature and prone to damage from the multitude of adverse medical complications to which these frail infants may be exposed. Lesions or atypical development of the prefrontal cortex occurring as a consequence of these hazardous events may have a detrimental effect on the development of EF which may have long-term consequences in terms of learning difficulties at school age. Indeed it has been found that children born preterm are at an increased risk for learning difficulties and attentional deficits when they reach school age and it has been suggested that this may be due to early abnormality in the development of the prefrontal cortex and consequently of executive dysfunction (16,17).

The ability to inhibit a prepotent response is also age-related, and like working memory, is first demonstrated at about 7-12 months of age (18), with improvements occurring between 18 and 30 months (19) in the primary school years (6-12 years) and again in young adults (18-29 years) (20).

Inhibition in children with learning difficulties and attention deficits

Barkley (2) described three components of inhibition, namely inhibition of a prepotent response, interruption of an ongoing response, and inhibition of interference from external stimuli. It has been found that children with learning difficulties also frequently have attention deficits (21). In a population-based epidemiological study, S.E. Shaywitz, B.A. Shaywitz,

Fletcher, and Escobar (22) found that 33% of children with learning difficulties also had attention deficits. Children with learning difficulties or attention deficits have been found consistently to have deficits in all three aspects of inhibition (23,24).

According to Barkley (2), deficient inhibition refers to impulsive acts or acting without thinking about the consequences. This impairs the ability of children with learning difficulties or attention deficits to engage in other appropriate and more timely activities. Consequently, these children miss out opportunities to learn.

Tasks assessing inhibition typically require an inappropriate response to be inhibited and irrelevant stimulus to be ignored. In a number of inhibition tasks such as the Go/No-Go task (24,25) and the Stroop Word-Color Test (23), children with learning difficulties showed poorer performance than typically developing children.

AB tasks

In addition to being able to mentally represent the object, the following abilities are required for infants to carry out the A*B* task successfully:

1. memory of the object's hiding location;
2. inhibition of the prepotent response to the previously correct location; and,
3. inhibition of interference from external stimuli (26).

Hence completion of this task clearly requires components of inhibition and it could therefore be regarded as a suitable means of assessing inhibition in human infants.

Inhibition of prepotent responses

Several researchers (27,28) have suggested that a combination of working memory deficits and inability to inhibit repetition of a previously rewarded response causes A*B* errors. Diamond suggested that the A*B* task sets up a conflict between the ability to use working memory to guide behaviour and a conditioned behavioural tendency to repeat a rewarded response when the object has been hidden at location B. Success at location A strengthens the tendency to reach to it by reinforcing this place response, and/or establishing a mental set for this response. The more frequently this response is reinforced the stronger the response tendency becomes. Infants of 8-12 months make A*B* errors because they fail to resist the 'reinforced habit' to repeat the previously successful responses at location A. This is evident from the study in which transparent occluders A and B were used, and infants still made A*B* errors although less frequently than when the occluders were opaque (29). Thus the learned habit seems at times to be stronger than even the attraction of the object.

Reaching to a previously rewarded location (location A) requires only working memory, but reaching to a new location (location B) requires both working memory and inhibition of the incorrect prepotent response, making the task more difficult and therefore more prone to errors. It is suggested that as the strength of the prepotent response increases due to repeated reinforcement, the ability to inhibit it must also increase if a correct response is to be made to a new location (30).

Inhibiting distraction from external stimuli

Interference control, or resistance to distraction, is defined by Barkley as the ability to "inhibit responding to sources of interference while engaged in another task requiring self-control or while delaying a response" (2). Whether or not distracters disrupt task performance depends upon the strength of the distracter and the potency of the response likely to be elicited by it (2). In the A*B* task, when a delay time is imposed between hiding and retrieval, external stimuli, such as the cover which is used to hide the object, may act as a distracter which interferes with the performance of the task. Few studies have, however, examined infants' ability to inhibit attention to distracter stimuli.

In summary, the analysis of performance on the A*B* task shows the importance of inhibition in completing this task. There is agreement that the inhibition abilities required to successfully carry out the A*B* task are working memory and inhibition of the prepotent response and consequently most studies have focused on these factors (27,31). It seems that inhibition to distraction from external stimuli is also required to conduct the A*B* task and few studies have examined this aspect of inhibition.

Previous research has shown that the general development of preterm infants occurs at a similar rate and follows a similar course to that of full-term infants when age is corrected for prematurity (32,33). This suggests that these basic patterns of development are predominantly governed by maturational factors. A number of people have argued that as developmental assessments are poor predictors of later learning abilities it is essential to assess more specific abilities (34) to improve the early identification of children who experience difficulties when they enter school. It is however not known whether these findings hold true for the development of specific cognitive abilities such as planning.

The development of inhibition was selected for investigation in the current study because these abilities are among the most significant cognitive achievements (35). Furthermore, inhibition deficits have been linked to learning problems which are particularly prevalent in preterm infants when they reach school age (36,37). The course of development of the inhibition in preterm infants remains unclear. As far as we know, the present report provides the first examination of the inhibition in preterm infants. The present study aimed to investigate this by comparing the performance of preterm and full-term infants on inhibition measure at the same corrected age and the same chronological age.

Our study

Participants in this study included a group of 37, eight month old preterm children born at ≤32 weeks gestation, and an age-matched group of 74 full-term control infants. Demographic information about the participating children is provided in Table 1. The research protocol was approved by the Human Research Ethics Committee at the Queensland University of Technology in Australia and informed parental consent was obtained for all mothers of participating infants. This study was conducted in conjunction with other research involving this group of infants (37,38). Recruitment procedures are described in detail in Sun et al (37,38).

Measurements

The Infant Working Memory and Inhibition task based on the A$\bar{B}$ task was arranged in degree of difficulty, in terms of the delay between hiding the object and being allowed to retrieve it, and the number of potential hiding places (cups). There were three levels of tasks (1-cup, 2-cup, and 3-cup tasks). There were three levels of delay (0, 4 and 10 s) for the 1-cup task and four levels of delay (0, 2, 4 and 10 s) for the 2-cup and 3-cup tasks. Thus there were a total of 11 conditions.

In the 1-cup task working memory for the object and inhibition to the distraction of the cup are needed to retrieve the goal object. In the 2-cup and 3-cup tasks working memory is needed to retrieve the goal object at location A and both working memory and inhibition are required in the changed location, that is location B. The Infant Working Memory and Inhibition task used in this study was therefore designed to measure working memory in the A positions, and inability to inhibit a prepotent response in the B positions in 2-cup and 3-cup tasks.

The materials used were 6 plastic cups with handles (1 yellow cup, 2 red cups, and 3 blue cups) which acted as occluders and 3 small round toys of different colours (red, yellow, and blue) which were selected following the pilot test (see section 5.3.3.4, and also Figure 5.1). The infants were asked to find the toy which they had seen being hidden underneath a cup.

According to Barkley (2), there are three components of inhibition, two of which were assessed in this study: (a) the ability to inhibit prepotent responses, and (b) interference control or resistance to distraction, which is the ability to inhibit interference from external environmental stimuli. Few studies on direct observation of the ability to inhibit interference from external stimuli in relation to EF tasks in infants could be located in the literature.

Scoring system for inhibition

Inhibition was assessed on the performances of the infants on the Infant Working Memory and Inhibition task described above. However, the scoring system used for inhibition was different from that used for working memory, thus enabling the separation of these two components of EF.

- The first component of inhibition (the ability to inhibit a prepotent response) occurs in conditions in which *conflicts* exist between responses that have a history of being reinforced, and responses which are required in the particular experimental condition. The A*B* task provides a condition in which response to the first hiding location (A) is repeated, then the hiding place changes from A to another location (B) which is identical to location A in appearance. In this situation infants have difficulty changing a previously reinforced response to location A, even when the occluder at that location is transparent and it is evident that there is no toy hidden there (29). It has been suggested that reaching to a new hiding position (B) is more difficult than to the previous hiding position (A), as reaching to B position requires infants both remembering the hiding location and inhibiting the incorrect reaching to A (27,39) (see table 5.2). It seems that the A*B* task creates a strong conflict between the previous response and the current response because the *incorrect*, impulsive response (reaching back to the previous hiding location) becomes prepotent. In the present study, the reinforcement to the previous hiding place was repeated once then changed to another location where there was an identical occluder. Therefore, scoring for inhibition of a prepotent response was based on infants' performance of incorrect reaching when the toy was changed to the B position in the 2-cup and 3-cup tasks (i.e., the 2nd, 4th, and 6th trials at each time delay level). In Table 5.2 these trials are printed in bold.

- The second aspect of inhibition, that of interference control or resistance to distraction, is the ability to inhibit responding to other sources of interference while engaged in the EF task or while delaying a response in the EF task. It has been found that the more salient the distraction, or the greater the time delays imposed within the task, the greater the likelihood that distracters will interfere with the task performance (2). In the current study, infants needed to inhibit inappropriate responses to the cup(s), for example playing with the cup(s) in order to retrieve the toy. Therefore, scoring for inhibition of distraction of external stimuli was based on infants' performance on distraction by the cups in 1-cup, 2-cup, and 3-cup tasks. Higher scores indicate greater inability to inhibit the distraction of the cups.

Perinatal variables: Medical complications, birthweight and gestation age

It is possible that some factors associated with being preterm affected performance of planning more than prematurity per se. These factors include medical complications, lower birthweight and shorter gestation age. Further analyses were conducted to assess the effect of perinatal variables which might have significantly affected preterm infants' performance on planning measures. For each of these factors the preterm infant group was divided into higher and lower risk groups, and the performance of each of these groups on planning measures was compared to that of the total full term infant group. Birthweight and gestation age were taken as separate factors in the analysis because there were eight preterm infants who were small for gestation age, therefore there was no correlation between birthweight and gestation age.

Preterm infants were firstly grouped on the basis of their severity of medical complication:

Demographic factors

Infants and their mothers were also assessed on the following confounding factors in the present study: infant motor and mental development, infant temperament, maternal education, family income, maternal psychological well-being.

Procedure

Mothers completed the background information form when the testing session was completed. Assessments for all infants were conducted in a testing room at Mater Children's Hospital. Infants and their mothers were videotaped as they participated in the planning tasks to permit later scoring of these tasks and the calculation of inter-rater reliability scores.

A familiarisation phase preceded testing sessions to enable each infant to become familiar with the experimenter and testing environment. In this phase, the infant was given a toy to play with for about two minutes. The experimenter described the study and gave instructions to the mother while the infant was playing. The mothers were instructed (a) not to give any help or clues to assist their infant's performance on any of the task, (b) to restrain baby's arms or body gently as instructed by the examiner during the delay time between hiding the object and when the infant was allowed to retrieve it in the working memory task, and (c) to ask for a break during the assessment if they felt it was necessary, for example, when the infant was hungry, sleepy, thirsty and so on. The mother was given time to feed the baby and change the infant's nappy before the assessment started.

Our findings

As there were no significant difference between preterm infants and full-term infants in demographic variables except psychomotor ability. Variable psychomotor ability was subsequently entered into Multivariate Analysis of Variance model to compare the difference between preterm and full-term infants in inhibition of prepotent response and inhibition to distraction of external stimuli.

Table 1 indicates that preterm infants had significantly lower score than full-term infants at both eight month and 10-11 months chronological age in two inhibition tasks between preterm infants and eight month full-term infants. Preterm infants has significantly lower scores than 10-11 month full-term infants in two inhibition tasks.

Table 1. Comparison between preterm and full-term infants at eight months corrected age and 10-11 month chronological age

Variables	Preterm group	Full-term (8 month)	Full term (10-11 months)	F	Posthoc
Inability to inhibit a prepotent response M (SD)	.48 (.20) A1	.31 (.16) A2	.25 (.14) A3	7.94***	A1 vs. A2*** (.00) A1 vs. A3*** (.00)
Inability to inhibit distraction M (SD)	.42 (.15) B1	.31 (.18) B2	.06 (.08) B3	42.63***	B1 vs. B2** (.01) B1 vs. B3*** (.00)

Note. 1. A1 to B3 are labels for ease of reporting comparisons between the means of three groups.
Preterm infant group: $n = 37$; Full-term infant group at eight month: $n = 74$;
Full-term infant group at 10-11 month chronological age: $n = 68$.
Posthoc test: Tukey's Honestly Significant Difference Test.
** $P < 0.01$, *** $P < 0.001$.

The findings in table 2 suggest that medical risk, lower birthweight, and lower gestation age adversely affect performance on inhibition measures. In each case, the high-risk group (i.e., the medical complications group, the <1,000 g birthweight group, and the < 28 weeks gestation group) performed more poorly than their low risk counterparts (i.e., the low medical risk group, the > 1,000 g birthweight group, and the > 28 weeks gestation group) on inhibition measures although these differences did not reach statistical significance.

The performance of both the high risk and low risk preterm groups on measures of inhibition were also consistently poorer than that of the full-term group, and this reached levels of statistical significance more frequently for the high risk preterm groups than for the low risk groups.

The results of the effects of perinatal factors on the performance of inhibition are summarised in table 2 below.

Table 2. Influence of perinatal risk factors on performance of executive function and sustained attention tasks when compared to full-term infants

Variables	Medical risk		Birthweight		Gestation age	
	High risk *p*	Low risk *p*	< 1000 g *p*	> 1000 g *p*	< 28 weeks *p*	> 28 weeks *p*
Inability to inhibit a prepotent response	.00***	.02*	NS	.00***	.00***	.00***
Inability to inhibit distraction	.00***	NS	NS	.01**	.06*	.05*

*Note.*The figures in the table above are summarised from Table 7.19, Table 7.20 and
Table 7.21 in section 7.6.3. NS means not statistically significant.
Significant difference between preterm infant group and full-term infant group:
p < .05, ** *p* < .01, *** *p* < .001.

Discussion

Findings in the present study are consistent with those of other researchers, who have reported that perinatal risk factors influence cognitive development during the first year of life (40-42).

Ross et al (42) for example reported high risk preterm infants showed lower scores on measures of working memory during infancy, but they did not examine inhibition as part of component of executive function which has been found in the present study. Similar deficits in executive function have also been reported in studies of school age children who were born preterm and who experienced high medical risk (17, 43). For example, Luciana et al (17) found that preterm born children at 7 to 9 years of age who had high medical risk differed from full-term infants on executive function tasks, and Taylor et al (44) also suggested that medical risk may influence the long term developmental outcomes of preterm infants.

The findings in the present study are also consistent with previous studies of children with extremely low birthweight, whether defined as birthweight < 1,000 g (16) or < 750 g (43), which have reported lower scores on the performance of inhibition tasks. However the children in these studies were older than the children in the present study. There is considerable evidence that tasks which require the inhibiting of a prepotent response involve the dorsolateral and ventro-lateral prefrontal cortex (45,46).

The deficits in all measures of inhibition observed in the high perinatal risk groups may be associated with the adverse effects of these perinatal risk factors on the prefrontal cortex which is very immature and sensitive in the preterm infants (47-49). Mouradian, Als and Coster (50) suggested that deficits in inhibition might be due to late maturing cortical organization, particularly of the prefrontal regions. Those preterm infants with these detrimental perinatal events are at particular risk for the abnormal prefrontal cortex functioning, hence the deficits in inhibition.

References

[1] Baddleley AD, Hitch G. Working memory. In: Bower GA, ed. Recent advances in learning and motivation. New York: Academic Press, 1974: 47-90.

[2] Barkley RA. Behavioral inhibition, sustained attention, and executive functions: Constructing a unifying theory of ADHD. Psychol Bull 1997;121(1):65-94.

[3] Mullen M, Snidman N, Kagan J. Free-play behavior in inhibited and uninhibited children. Infant Behav Dev 1993;16:383-9.

[4] Kerr M, Lambert WW. Stability of inhibition in a Swedish longitudinal sample. Child Dev 1994;65:138-46.

[5] Calkins SD, Fox NA, Marshall TR. Behavioral and physiological antecedents of inhibited and uninhibited behavior. Child Dev 1996;67:523-40.

[6] Fuster JM. The prefrontal cortex: Anatomy, physiology, and neuropsychology of the frontal lobe. New York: Lippincott-Raven; 1997.

[7] Lezak MD. The problem of assessing executive functions. Int J Psychol 1982;17:281-97.

[8] Milner B. Effects of different brain lesions on card sorting. Arch Neurol 1963;9:90-100.

[9] Chao LL, Knight RT. Human prefrontal lesions increase distractibility to irrelevant sensory inputs. NeuroReport 1995;6:1605-10.

[10] Stuss DT. Interference effects on memory functions in postleukotomy patients: An attentional perspective. In: Levin HS, Eisenberg HM, Benton AL, eds. Frontal lobe function and dysfunction. New York: Oxford University Press, 1991:157-72.

[11] Fuster JM. Role of prefrontal cortex in delay tasks: Evidence from reversible lesion and unit recording in the monkey. In: Levin HS, Eisenberg HM, eds. Frontal function and dysfunction. New York: Oxford University Press, 1991:59-71.

[12] Goldman-Rakic PS, Rosvold HE. The effects of selective caudate lesions in infant and juvenile rhesus monkeys. Brain Res 1972;42:53-66.

[13] Kubota K. Delayed response and perseverative errors in newborn infant rhesus monkeys. In: Ono T, Squire LR, Raichle ME, Perrett DI, Fukuda M, eds. Brain mechamisms of perception and memory: From neuron to behavior. New York: Oxford University Press, 1993:457-63.

[14] Goldman-Rakic PS. Development of cortical circuitry and cognitive function. Child Dev 1987;58:601-22.

[15] Thatcher RW. Maturation of the human frontal lobes: Physiological evidence for staging. Dev Neuropsychol 1991;7(3):397-419.

[16] Harvey JM, O'Callaghan MJ, Mohay H. Executive function of children with extremely low birthweight: A case control study. Dev Med Child Neurol 1999;41:292-7.

[17] Luciana M, Lindeke L, Georgieff M, Mills M, Nelson CA. Neurobehavioral evidence for working-memory deficits in school-aged children with histories of prematurity. Dev Med Child Neurol 1999;41:521-33.

[18] Diamond A, Doar B. The performance of human infants on a measure of frontal cortex function, the delayed response task. Dev Psychobiol 1989;22(3):271-94.

[19] Vaughn BE, Kopp CB, Krakow JB. The emergence and consolidation of self-control from eighteen to thirty months of age: Normative trends and individual differences. Child Dev 1984;55:990-1004.

[20] Williams BR, Ponesse JS, Schachar RJ, Logan GD, Tannock R. Development of inhibitory control across the life span. Dev Psychol 1999;35(1):205-13.

[21] Barkley RA, Grodzinsky GM. Are tests of frontal lobe functions useful in the diagnosis of attention-deficit disorders? Clin Neuropsychol 1994;8(2):121-39.

[22] Shaywitz SE, Shaywitz BA, Fletcher JM, Escobar MD. Prevalence of reading disability in boys and girls. JAMA 1990;264:998-1002.

[23] Pennington BF, Groisser D, Welsh MC. Contrasting cognitive deficits in attention deficit hyperactivity disorder versus reading disability. Dev Psychol 1993;29(3):511-23.

[24] Schachar R, Mota VL, Logan GD, Tannock R, Klim P. Confirmation of an inhibitory control deficit in attention-deficit/hyperactivity disorder. J Abnorm Child Psychol 2000;28(3):227-35.

[25] Nigg JT. The ADHD response-inhibition deficit as measured by the stop task: Replication with DSM-IV combined type, extension, and qualification. J Abnorm Child Psychol 1999;27(5):393-402.

[26] Diamond A. The development and neural bases of memory functions as indexed by the A*B* and delayed response tasks in human infants and infant monkeys. The development and neural bases of higher cognitive functions: Annals of the New York Academy of Sciences. New York: New York Academy Sciences, 1990: 394-433.

[27] Diamond A. Abilities and neural mechanisms underlying A*B* performance. Child Dev 1988;59:523-7.

[28] McCall DD, Clifton RK. Infants' means-end search for hidden objects in the absence of visual feedback. Infant Behav Dev 1999;22:179-95.

[29] Butterworth G. Object disappearance and error in Piaget's stage IV task. J Exp Child Psychol 1977;23:391-401.

[30] Diamond A, Werker JF, Lalonde C. Toward understanding commonalities in the development of object search, detour navigation, categorization, and speech perception. In: Dawson G, Fischer KW, eds. Human behavior and the developing brain. New York: Guilford , 1994:380-426.

[31] Diamond A. Development of the ability to use recall to guide action, as indicated by infants' performance on A*B*. Child Dev 1985;56:868-83.

[32] Ross G, Lipper E, Auld PAM. Cognitive abilities and early precursors of learning disabilities in very-low-birthweight children with normal intelligence and normal neurological status. Int J Behav Dev 1996;19(3):563-80.

[33] Rutter M. Developing minds: Challenge and continuity across the life span. London, England: Penguin; 1992.

[34] McCall RB. What process mediates predictions of childhood IQ from infant habituation and recognition memory? Speculations on the roles of inhibition and rate of information processing. Intelligence 1994;18:107-25.

[35] Aron A, Robbins TW, Poldrack RA. Inhibition and the right inferior frontal cortex. Trends Cogn Sci 2004;8(4):172-7.

[36] Halari R, Simic M, Pariante CM, Papadopoulos A, Cleare A, Brammer M, et al. Reduced activation in lateral prefrontal cortex and anterior cingulate during attention and cognitive control functions in medication-naïve adolescents with depression compared to controls. J Child Psychol Psychiatry 2009;50(3):307-16.

[37] Sun J, Mohay H, O'Callaghan M. Executive function in preterm and full-term infants. Early Hum Dev 2009;85(4):225-30.

[38] Sun J, Buys N. Prefrontal lobe functioning and its relationship to working memory in preterm infants. Int J Child Adolesc Health 2011;4(1):13-7.

[39] Harris PL. Perseverative errors in search by young infants. Child Dev 1973;44: 28-33.

[40] Molfese V, Thomson B. Optimality versus complications: Assessing predictive values of perinatal scales. Child Dev 1985;56:810-23.

[41] Piper MC, Kunos I, Willis DM, Mazer B. Effect of gestational age on neurological functioning of the very low-birthweight infant at 40 weeks. Dev Med Child Neurol 1985;27:596-605.

[42] Ross G, Tesman J, Auld PM, Nass R. Effects of subependymal and mild intraventricular lesions on visual attention and memory in premature infants. Dev Psychol 1992;28(6):1067-74.

[43] Taylor HG, Klein N, Minich NM, Hack M. Middle-school-age outcomes in children with very low birthweight. Child Dev 2000;71:1495-511.

[44] Taylor HG, Klein N, Schatschneider C, Hack M. Predictors of early school age outcomes in very low birth weight children. Dev Behav Pediatr 1998;19(4):235-43.

[45] Diamond A, Kirkham N, Amso D. Conditions under which young children can hold two rules in mind and inhibit a prepotent response. Dev Psychol 2002;38(3):352-62.

[46] Roberts JRJ, Pennington BF. An interactive framework for examining prefrontal cognitive processes. Dev Neuropsychol 1996;12(1):105-26.

[47] Aylward GP. Perinatal asphyxia: Effects of biological and environmental risks. Clin Perinat 1993;20:433-49.

[48] Diamond A, Lee E. Inability of five-month-old infants to retrieve a contiguous object: A failure of conceptual understanding or of control of action? Child Dev 2000;71(6):1477-94.

[49] Fletcher JM, Brookshire BL, Landry SH, Bohan TP, Davidson KC, Francis DJ, et al. Attentional skills and executive functions in children with early hydrocephalus. Dev Neuropsychol 1996;12(1):53-76.

[50] Mouradian LE, Als H, Coster WJ. Neurobehavioral functioning of healthy preterm infants of varying gestational ages. Dev Behav Pediatr 2000;21(6):408-16.

Chapter III

Executive function and general development in preterm and full-term infants

Abstract

This chapter investigates the relationship between executive function and general development in preterm at eight months corrected age and full-term infants at eight months. The assessment of subtle developmental and behavioural delays in infants is complicated, and currently there are few sensitive measures available for the early identification of learning problems in infants. Conventional developmental assessment tools, for example, the Bayley Scales of Infant Development, only provide global indicators of development and fail to measure specific skills that may provide sensitive predictions of later learning. The assessment of specific cognitive skills, such as executive function (EF) rather than a global development score in infancy, has been advocated by a number of investigators Thirty-seven preterm infants without identified disabilities, and 74 due date and gender matched healthy full-term infants, participated in the present study. The preterm infants were all less than 32 weeks gestation and less than 1,500 grams birthweight. All infants were therefore assessed on general development, working memory, inhibition to prepotent response and inhibitioni to distraction of external stimuli, and planning tasks at 8 months after the expected date of delivery. The findings of the study showed EF was not correlated with either motor or mental scores of Bayley Infant Development Assessment. The results of this study suggests that the EF is independent of general abilities as assessed by Bayley Scales of Infant Development.

Introduction

Infant assessment instruments such as the Bayley Scales of Infant Development (1) have been used frequently as early outcome measures in studies monitoring the development of preterm infants (2-4). They have also been used as predictors of long-term developmental outcomes. Measures of general development in infancy, such as the Bayley Scales of Infant Development (1), have been found to be poor predictors of developmental outcomes in childhood, even for high-risk groups (5,6). This is partly due to the fact that most of the items in these infant measures reflect sensorimotor development, and are therefore qualitatively different from achievements in abstract, verbal, and symbolic reasoning which are assessed on intelligence and achievement tests for older children. Furthermore, traditional infant developmental tests provide a view of cognitive development only in the context of the infant's overall developmental level, although an individual may be performing at different levels in different skill areas. A composite score cannot capture patterns of strengths and weaknesses in such areas as vocabulary knowledge, memory, logical thinking and spatial abilities that may underlie later learning problems.

Measures of specific abilities: Executive function (EF)

A number of different research strategies have been used to study more subtle measures of specific abilities. These include paradigms such as Piaget's A*B* task and infant planning tasks. A number of investigators have examined paradigms that focus on infants' actions on objects as strategies for identifying what might be long term cognitive deficits. From a neuropsychological perspective, recent research has suggested that performance on tasks such as the A*B* task and planning tasks are linked to the development of executive function in infants (7,8). These measures may therefore be sufficiently sensitive to predict later development, when they are interpreted in terms of the development of the EF abilities which are believed to underlie learning (9-12).

Until the 1980s it had been thought that the frontal lobes were dormant during infancy and that EF could therefore not be measured. However, evidence has emerged to show that the frontal lobes are active and that EF arises in infancy (13). Studies using the A*B* task have demonstrated that at around 7-8 months, infants begin to understand that an object continues to exist even when out of sight. Reaching to the correct position in the A*B* task requires infants to hold information in mind to guide the correct response. This requires working memory. Infants at this age (i.e., 7-8 months) have also been shown to be able to sequence steps and achieve a goal, which requires planning ability (14) and therefore similarly suggests that EF must be operating. A number of investigators have proposed that learning difficulties and attentional deficits frequently identified in children born preterm may be linked to the impairment of one or more components of EF (15, 16), such as planning, working memory and inhibition. A detailed discussion about the concept of EF and SA, its relation to learning and brain function, and the pattern of development and measurement of EF.

EF is a general term. It is a complex abstract concept associated with a wide range of higher-order cognitive functions and a variety of behaviours (for more detail, see 17). It has been shown to be related to cognitive development and learning in the following ways:

- as a control process for the organisation of behaviour (18);
- as a component of higher-order cognitive functioning (19); and,
- as a regulator of behaviours which contribute to flexible and fluid intellectual functioning (20).

EF is deliberate, conscious, and purposeful (21,22). The neuro-psychological perspective adopted by Stuss (22) emphasised that EF does not belong with elementary cognitive processes, such as perception and memory, but is associated with higher-order cognitive abilities, including working memory, inhibition, planning and so forth. At EF level, cognition is deliberate and effortful and is required for the processing of new or complex material where routine responses or knowledge are not effective (21). With repetition, the new complex behaviours requiring active conscious deliberation may eventually become automatic and are then transferred to a lower cognitive level (22). The distinction between higher and lower levels of cognition is determined by the degree of "mental effort" required to carry out a particular task (21). Rabbitt for example described EF as

    . . . necessary to deal with novel tasks that require us to formulate a goal, to plan and to choose between alternative sequences of behaviour to reach this goal, to compare these plans in respect of their relative probabilities of success and their relative efficiency in attaining the chosen goal, to initiate the plan selected and to carry it through, amending it as necessary, until it is successful or until impending failure is recognised (21)

EF is a control process which requires recognition, evaluation, and choice among a variety of alternative options and strategies, whereas non-EF processes are automatic and do not require consideration or evaluation of alternative strategies. EF is operating in the early stages of learning a new skill (e.g., thinking about what one is doing). However, once a task has become routine (after much practice), EF is not required for execution of the skill and one no longer has to think about what he/she is doing.

Studying a group of infants at high-risk for learning difficulties should make it easier to identify factors that are predictive of later learning problems. This may lead to a greater understanding of the etiology of these problems in all children. The relationship between EF and general development in infancy, such as the Bayley Scales of Infant Development, has not been studied. The present study aimed to examine the relationship btween EF and scores on the Bayley Scales of Infant Development in preterm and full-term infants.

The research questions were: Do the scores on the measures of EF correlate with the scores on the Bayley Scales of Infant Development?

Our study

All subjects were recruited through the Mater Children's Hospital, Brisbane where they were all born. Both preterm and full-term infants were healthy and without any. There were 37 preterm infants with birthweights of < 1500 g and < 28 weeks gestation and 74 full-term infants with normal birhtweight and gestational age and no medical complications in the perinatal period participated in the study. Full-term infants were matched to preterm infants in age and gender. Details of the participants were described in published literature (23,24)

Infants and their mothers were also assessed on the infant motor and mental development, working memory, inhibition and planning. All infants were assessed on the above variables at 8 months after the expected date of delivery (preterm infants were 10 to 11 months chronological age at this time). The characteristics of the participants can be found in the published papers (24).

The Bayley Scales of Infant Development (2nd edition) (1) were used to provide a standard measure of infant development. This test has been widely used in a number of studies (2-4) and has acceptable psychometric properties. It provides separate assessments for Mental development (MDI) and Motor Development (PDI). The MDI includes items that assess memory, habituation, vocalisation, language and social skills. The examples of the items include: retains two cubes for 3 seconds, manipulates bell showing interest in detail, attends to scribbling, vocalises three different vowel sounds, pulls string adaptively to secure ring, and so forth. The PDI assesses the ability to control the gross and fine muscle groups. This includes movement associated with rolling, crawling and creeping, sitting, standing, and walking. Fine motor skills including prehension and manipulation of objects. The examples of the items for fine motor skills include: uses partial thumb opposition to grasp pellet, uses pades of fingertips to grasp pellet, etc. All raw scores were converted to index scores based on corrected age for preterm infants. The MDI was used to exclude children from the study who had delayed general development. Although EF and SA have generally been regarded as independent of general development, it was felt important to ensure that scores of general development were within average range especially as numerous studies have shown the development of preterm infants to be somewhat behind that of term infants (25, 26).

EF was assessed by Infant Working Memory and Inhibition tasks and planning tasks (24). To answer these research questions, Pearson's product-moment correlation was used to analyse the relationship between performance on the different components of EF, SA, and general development for preterm and the full-term infants groups and a correlation matrix generated. Because of the large number of variables included in the analysis there is an increased chance of false positive results. Therefore it was decided to consider only correlations between variables which reached a significance level $p < .01$.

What we found

Table 1 shows that when only infants with PDI above 85 were included in the analysis, the pattern of the relationship was similar for both the preterm and full-term infants. That is, most EF measures did not correlate with each other, and Bayley PDI and MDI did not correlate with either EF measures.

Table 1. A correlations matrix among the variables of working memory, inhibition, planning, general development and sustained attention for preterm (n = 29) and full-term infants (n = 73) with the exclusion of infants with Bayley PDI less than 85

	Working Memory	Inhibit Prepotent response	Inhibit Distrac	Planning	MDI	PDI
Executive function 1.Working Memory Full-term infants	1.00					
Preterm infants	1.00					
2. Inability to inhibit prepotent response Full-term infants	-.23 (.04)	1.00				
Preterm Infants	-.46 (.01)	1.00				
3. Inability to inhibit distraction Full-term infants	-.23 (.04)	.08 (.51)	1.00			
Preterm infants	-.07 (.71)	.07 (.72)	1.00			
4. Planning Full-term infants	.09 (.47)	.07 (.55)	.03 (.77)	1.00		
Preterm infants	.20 (.29)	-.38 (.04)	-.34 (.07)	1.00		
Bayley Scores 1. Bayley MDI Full-term infants	.23 (.05)	-.08 (.50)	-.21 (.06)	.16 (.16)	1.00	
Preterm infants	.30 (.11)	-.29 (.13)	.18 (.35)	.28 (.15)	1.00	
2. Bayley PDI Full-term infants	.28 (.02)	-.003 (.97)	- .15 (.20)	.22 (.06)	.39 (.00)	1.00
Preterm infants	.38 (.04)	-.37 (.05)	-.02 (.93)	.29 (.13)	.47 (.01)	1.00

The findings suggest that measures of EF may be discrete abilities and that EF is independent of infant general development.

When the infants scoring below 85 on PDI were removed from the analysis, the relationships between the following variables for preterm infants showed different results than before the infants were removed: (a) Bayley PDI and working memory, (b) Bayley PDI and inability to inhibit a prepotent response, (c) planning and inability to inhibit a prepotent response. These findings confirmed the finding that the delayed psychomotor development in some preterm infants significantly influenced the performance of working memory, inability to inhibit a prepotent response, and planning of EF in the preterm infant group.

As the level of the significant correlation between working memory and inability to inhibit a prepotent response in preterm infants ($r = -.46$) is similar to full-term infants ($r = -.23$), the significant correlation between these two variables in preterm infants may disappear if the number of preterm infants is increased.

Discussion

There were no significant correlations between Bayley PDI or MDI and any measures of EF when infants with PDI scores < 85 were excluded. This suggests that for infants who are functioning within or above the average range, EF and general development are independent. This is consistent with the findings from studies of older children and adults (27, 28). When infants with low Bayley PDI scores were included in the analysis there was a significant correlation between (1) PDI scores and both working memory and inability to inhibit a prepotent response for preterm infants, and (2) between PDI and working memory for full-term infants. These findings suggest that low Bayley PDI scores influence performance on EF tasks, however it is impossible to tell whether poor motor skills interfere with the actual development of EF.

The components of EF did not correlate with with general development. All of these findings have significant theoretical and practical implications for future research and clinical practice. Previous studies (14, 29, 30) have focused on only one or at most two aspects of EF, and thus provided a more restricted view of these abilities and their relationship to other cognitive processes in infancy.

In order to carry out such a broad-ranging project it was necessary to design and/or modify existing tests of EF. The results indicate that it is not only possible to measure EF in infancy, but as preterm infants were found to show inferior performances on the EF, it is also possible to detect deficits in EF in infants who are at high-risk for later learning difficulties and attentional deficits.

References

[1] Bayley N. Bayley scale of infant development: Manual, 2nd ed. San Antonio, TX: Psychological Corporation, 1993.

[2] Hack M, Friedman H, Fanaroff AA. Outcomes of extremely low birth weight infants. Pediatrics 1996;98(5):931-7.

[3] O'Shea TM, Klinepeter L, Goldstein DJ, Jackson BW, Dillard RG. Survival and developmental disability in infants with birth weights of 501 to 800 grams, born between 1979 and 1994. Pediatrics 1997;100(6):982-6.

[4] Vohr BR, Wright LL, Dusick AM, Mele L, Verter J, Steichen JJ, et al. Neurodevelopmental and functional outcomes of extremely low birth weight infants in the National Institute of Child Health and Human Development neonatal research network, 1993-1994. Pediatrics 2000;105(6):1216-26.

[5] Aylward GP, Pfeiffer SI, Wright A, Verhulst SJ. Outcome studies of low birth weight infants published in the last decade: A meta-analysis. J Pediatr 1989;115:515-20.

[6] Siegel LS. IQ is irrelevant to the definition of learning disabilities. J Learn Disabil 1989;22(8):469-78.

[7] Bell MA, Fox NA. The relations between frontal brain electrical activity and cognitive development during infancy. Child Dev 1992;63:1142-63.

[8] Diamond A. Abilities and neural mechanisms underlying AB performance. Child Dev 1988;59:523-7.

[9] Adams JW, Snowling MJ. Executive function and reading impairments in children reported by their teachers as 'hyperactive'. Br J Dev Psychol 2001;19:293-306.

[10] Denckla MB. Biological correlates of learning and attention: What is relevant to learning disabilities and attention-deficit hyperactivity disorder? Dev Behav Pediatr 1996;17(2):114-9.

[11] Passolunghi MC, Siegel LS. Short-term memory, working memory, and inhibitory control in children with difficulties in arithmetic problem solving. J Exp Child Psychol 2001;80:44-57.

[12] Snow JH. Developmental patterns and use of the Wisconsin Card Sorting Test for children and adolescents with learning disabilities. Child Neuropsychol 1998;4(2):89-97.

[13] Diamond A. Development of the ability to use recall to guide action, as indicated by infants' performance on AB. Child Dev 1985;56:868-83.

[14] Willatts P. Development of means-end behavior in young infants: Pulling a support to retrieve a distant object. Dev Psychol 1999;35(3):651-67.

[15] Gathercole SE. The development of memory. J Child Psychol Psychiatry 1998;39(1):3-27.

[16] Luciana M, Lindeke L, Georgieff M, Mills M, Nelson CA. Neurobehavioral evidence for working-memory deficits in school-aged children with histories of prematurity. Dev Med Child Neurol 1999;41:521-33.

[17] Lyon GR, Krasnegor NA. Attention, memory and executive function. Baltimore, MD: Paul H Brookes, 1996.

[18] Borskowski JG, Burke JE. Theories, models, and measurement of executive functioning: An information processing perspective. In: Lyon GR, Krasnegor NA, editors. Attention, memory, and executive function. Baltimore, MD: Paul H Brookes, 1996:235-61.

[19] Stuss DT, Eskes GA, Foster JK. Experimental neuropsychological studies of frontal lobe functions. In: Boller F, Spinnler H, Hendler JA, editors. Handbook of neuropsychology. Amsterdam: Elsevier, 1994:149-85.

[20] Burgess PW. Theory and methodology in executive function research. In: Rabbitt P, editor. Methodology of frontal and executive function. Hove, East Sussex: Psychology Press, 1997:81-116.

[21] Rabbitt P. Introduction: Methodologies and models in the study of executive function. In: Rabbitt P, ed. Methodology of frontal and executive function. Hove, East Sussex: Psychology Press, 1997:1-38.

[22] Stuss DT. Biological and psychological development of executive functions. Brain Cogn 1992;20:8-23.

[23] Sun J, Buys N. Prefrontal lobe functioning and its relationship to working memory in preterm infants. Int J Child Adolesc Health 2011;4(1):13-7.

[24] Sun J, Mohay H, O'Callaghan M. Executive function in preterm and full-term infants. Early Hum Dev 2009;85(4):225-30.

[25] Landry SH, Chapieski ML. Visual attention during toy exploration in preterm infants: Effects of medical risk and maternal interactions. Infant Behav Dev 1988;11:187-204.

[26] Rose SA, Feldman JF, Wallace IF, McCarton C. Infant visual attention: Relation to birth status and developmental outcome during the first 5 years. Dev Psychol 1989;25(4):560-76.

[27] Ardila A, Pineda D, Rosselli M. Correlation between intelligence test scores and executive function measures. Arch Clin Neuropsychol 2000;15(1):31-6.

[28] Welsh MC, Pennington BF, Groisser DB. A normative-developmental study of executive function: A window on prefrontal function in children. Dev Neuropsychol 1991;7(2):131-49.

[29] Diamond A, Doar B. The performance of human infants on a measure of frontal cortex function, the delayed response task. Dev Psychobiol 1989;22(3):271-94.

[30] Diamond A, Gilbert J. Development as progressive inhibitory control of action: Retrieval of a contiguous object. Cogn Dev 1989;4:223-49.

Chapter IV

Planning and prefrontal lobe functioning in preterm and full term infants

Abstract

This chapter investigatesplanning in preterm and full-term infants at eight months after expected date of delivery. Planning emerges in infancy and continues to develop throughout childhood. Planning is believed to underlie some learning problems in children at school age. This study investigated planning in preterm and full-term infants at eight months after expected date of delivery. Thirty-seven preterm infants without identified disabilities, and 74 due date and gender matched healthy full-term infants, participated in the present study. The preterm infants were all less than 32 weeks gestation and less than 1,500 grams birthweight. All infants were therefore assessed on planning tasks at 8 months after the expected date of delivery (when preterm infants were actually 10-11 months chronological age). The findings of the study showed that preterm infants performed significantly more poorly than full-term infants at both eight months corrected age and 10-11 month chronological age on measures of in one-step, three steps, four steps and five steps planning tasks, but not in two-step task. Medical risk, lower birthweight and lower gestation age were found significantly affect the performance on planning tasks. The findings of this study suggests that the deficits of planning in preterm infants may be associated with lower birthweight, shorter gestatation and medical complications which may have further detrimental effect.

Introduction

Planning is purposive and goal directed (1). Planning requires generating novel, complex and hierarchically organised behaviour in order to attain a goal (2-4). Planning involves several core concepts, such as intention, sequencing of actions, and strategies (2,3). Intention is deliberate and includes "conscious representation of a goal, the active consideration of alternative means and ends, and the feeling accompanying the selection and execution of a plan" (5). Planning may involve a sequence of actions that act as a bridge between the intention and the goal (6-8). This demands that the individual be adaptable and flexible in the face of changing circumstances in order to modify and redirect the original plan (4,9). Planning involves strategy analysis, which serves to organise past knowledge, new information and actions (2,10). The planner needs to foresee that the goal state can not be achieved directly, but that a series of sub-goals, or steps, reduces the distance between the current position and the goal state (10). Means-ends analysis can be applied from the initial state of the problem through the selection of a set of operations that will construct a path from this state to the goal state (2).

Planning requires subjects to keep track of their intention or goal, formulate the sequence of actions and then when possible carry out the plan. By definition, planning involves situations for which the individual has no readily available response and which require the generation of a novel response to reach a goal (9). From an information-processing perspective, planning involves five operations: (a) representing the problem, (b) setting the goal, (c) building a strategy, (d) executing the plan, and (e) monitoring and repairing (11), which are necessary steps to complete a planning task. Execution of the plan is a necessary step to achieving a goal. From a cognitive perpective, Willatts (2) suggested that planning tasks involving means-end problem solving which is intentionally planned with a goal in mind. This includes mentally representing the goal, identifying the subgoal (such as two-step task), and finding the solution in advance of any action and without feedback. According to Willatts and Rosie (6), the solution of the problem may be planned in advance but may not be executed.

Tasks assessing planning typically require a sequence of steps to be planned, monitored and revised in advance of actions executed. For example, the Tower of Hanoi and Tower of London tasks require that a set of discs or balls placed on one peg (a start state), be reproduced on a different peg (the goal state) in the fewest moves possible. Both the Tower of Hanoi and the

Tower of London impose a set of rules that constrain the manner in which the objects may be moved from peg to peg, although the rules differ somewhat between the two tasks. Based on these rules and the structure of the Tower of Hanoi and the Tower of London tasks, successful performance requires a sequence of moves to be planned, executed, monitored, and revised. From an initial position of the balls on the sticks (for example, red over green on the long stick, and blue on the middle stick), the subject is asked to move balls from stick to stick to achieve a certain display in a specified number of moves (for example, green over blue over red on the long stick in five moves). In order to reach the goal-state the subject must plan and execute a series of steps in the proper sequence. The tower tasks have been used to assess planning abilities of typical children and adults, children and adults with intellectual impairment (12), and adults with frontal damage (13,14). The research found that the performance on the tasks distinguished children with abnormal development from typically developing children (15).

The failure to formulate a plan to attain a goal, especially in a new situation, is generally accepted as a common feature of executive dysfunction associated with clinical damage to the prefrontal cortex (16,17). The successful execution of a plan necessitates a prior conceptual scheme of the plan, the preparation for each of the steps to implement it, and the anticipation of attaining the goal. It is difficult for frontal patients to plan due to their poor anticipation or inability to execute a sequence of actions.

The difficulties experienced by frontal patients in organising behavioural sequences have been demonstrated on a large number of neuropsychological tests that require temporal ordering, learning of new skills, monitoring the temporal sequence of events, or the execution of a series of actions (16). Patients with damage to the prefrontal cortex have no trouble executing old and well-rehearsed routines, but encounter difficulty when forced to develop a new form of behaviour based on deliberation and choice, especially if in order to reach the goal it is necessary to organise a novel sequence of acts or a new plan (14).

Regardless of the lesion site, the frontal patient's difficulty in organising behaviour is only evident in challenging situations and may not surface in everyday life (16,18,19). The severity of the disorder may vary considerably. In many patients, the disorder is not incompatible with ordinary life, especially if the lesion is in the dorsolateral region, which is related to planning ability. The patient's life may become more ordinary and ordered than it would normally be, and troubles may appear only when the patient is confronted with new challenges or changes in the environment (17,20).

Defective planning is particularly evident on tasks that require internal planning of new behaviour (21,22). For example, the Tower of Hanoi has been considered a test of planning, and has been used with patients who have frontal lobe damage (14). These patients, especially those with damage to the left hemisphere, have been found to be severely impaired in performance on the Tower of London task (23,24). The ability to plan and execute schemes of action is adversely affected when frontal lobe lesions occur, especially if these are in the left dorsolateral prefrontal cortex. Hence frontal patients commonly show difficulties in the initiation and organisation of new behaviour.

Willatts (2) found that planning ability similarly emerges in infants at 7-8 months of age, and Chen, Sanchez and Campbell (25) showed that children at 13 months of age were able to plan and execute the necessary course of action to solve age-appropriate problems and use flexibility in the choice of strategies to solve the problems. Bauer et al (4) reported that at 18 to 27 months of age children had developed the ability to represent the goal state of a problem and to plan, monitor, and execute a course of action necessary to achieve it. The planning tasks used with children under two years of age typically require them to remove an obstacle to attain a goal. Older children are usually required to generate a path to a goal. For example, the Tower of Hanoi, which requires children to plan a course of action to reach the goal state, has been used with children from 3 years of age, with marked improvements in performance being observed from the ages of three to twelve, when adult levels of performance are achieved (26,27).

Previous research has shown that the general development of preterm infants occurs at a similar rate and follows a similar course to that of full-term infants when age is corrected for prematurity (28,29). This suggests that these basic patterns of development are predominantly governed by maturational factors. A number of people have argued that as developmental assessments are poor predictors of later learning abilities it is essential to assess more specific abilities (30) to improve the early identification of children who experience difficulties when they enter school. It is however not known whether these findings hold true for the development of specific cognitive abilities such as planning.

The development of planning was selected for investigation in the current study because these abilities are among the most significant cognitive achievements (2). Furthermore, planning deficits have been linked to learning problems which are particularly prevalent in preterm infants when they reach school age (31,32). The course of development of the planning in preterm infants remains unclear. As far as we know, the present report provides the first examination of the planning in preterm infants. The present study aimed to investigate this by comparing the performance of preterm and full-term infants on planning measure at the same corrected age and the same chronological age.

Our study

Participants in this study included a group of 37, eight month old preterm children born at ≤32 weeks gestation, and an age-matched group of 74 full-term control infants. Demographic information about the participating children is provided in Table 1a. The research protocol was approved by the Human Research Ethics Committee at the Queensland University of Technology in Australia and informed parental consent was obtained for all mothers of participating infants. This study was conducted in conjunction with other research involving this group of infants (33,34). Recruitment procedures are described in detail in Sun et al (33, 34).

The planning tasks previously utilised in a number of studies (2,35-37) were modified for use in the current study. The following factors were taken into consideration in the design of the planning task.

1. The age of the child. The tasks must be suitable to children at 8-12 months. At this age infants have developed the necessary motor skills for reaching, pulling, grasping, and lifting, therefore these skills can constitute the responses required in a planning task (38).

2. The difficulty of the task. The difficulty of the task must increase progressively in order to avoid basal and ceiling problems. At the simplest level, eight-month-old infants must be able to pass some items and at the most difficult level the tasks must be challenging for 12-month-old infants. The difficulty of the task is influenced by the following factors:

   a. The number of steps required to reach the goal. In Willatts' studies for infants from 7 months to 12 months of age, he found that at eight months of age infants could solve a 1-step cloth-support problem , that is, pulling a cloth to retrieve an object that was resting on it (2). At nine months they could solve a 2-step planning task, which involved removing a barrier, then pulling a cloth to retrieve an object that was resting on it (36). At 12 months of age, they could carry out a three-step planning task to obtain a goal (37), which involved removing a barrier, then pulling a cloth which was used to cover the toy, and finally removing the cloth to get the toy. In the current study, the problems presented to the infants progressively increased in difficulty from one step to five steps, so that they were required to construct increasingly longer sequences of actions in order to reach a goal.

b. The directness/indirectness of the route to the goal. In the design of the planning task, Willatts and Rosie (6) suggested that the principle of the planning task was to overcome obstacles along an existing path to a desired goal. The route to the desired goal in this case was direct. For example, when the goal toy was resting on a cloth which needed to be pulled in order to retrieve the toy, the route was perceivable and there were no alternatives (i.e., no choices have to be made). An indirect route to the goal makes the task more difficult as choices between alternative actions have to be made at various points along the route to the goal. For example, the child may have to choose to pull one of two strings, only one of which is attached to the desired toy. Chen, Sanchez, and Campbell (25) argued that infants from 10 to 13 months of age could solve more difficult tasks than in Willatts et al.'s study (6, 37) and used a task involving an indirect route to the goal. In their planning task a barrier was put in front of two pieces of cloth, each of which had a string on it. A toy was attached to one string but not to the other. The task was therefore more complex as the infants were required to decide which string was attached to the toy, and then to pull the appropriate cloth in order to get the right string and hence the toy. The choices between two routes had to be made, thus requiring advanced planning of the route to get to the goal.

c. The arrangement of means-end problems. In means-end problems, the means are methods to attain a goal. A sequence of subgoals needs to be attained in order to reach the goal. In Willatts'(39) 3-step task the subgoals were (a) to get the cloth (by removing the barrier), (b) to get the string (by pulling the cloth) and (c) to get the toy. The subgoals (a) and (b) have to be attained before the toy can be retrieved.

In the current study, the 1-step, 2-step, and 3-step tasks were utilised. The tasks were similar to planning tasks used in previous studies (2, 36, 37), except that the barrier was transparent allowing the goal object to be visible at all times. In a 4-step task, which was designed specifically for this study, the first three steps were the same as above and a Perspex box which had to be removed by the infant was used to cover the toy. A 5-step task actually requires four steps to get the toy. It is called 5-step task as the task is more difficult than the 4-step task because it changes from a direct path to an indirect path to the goal. The 5-step task was similar to Chen et al.'s (25) study, in which two cloths and strings were used; however it was different from Chen et al. because two toys rather than one were used, with only one toy being attached to a string. It seems uncessary to have two toys as the toy which was attached with the string that was rested on the cloth is determined by the cloth step. That is, the infants had to choose between two cloths in constructing a plan to reach the toy.

Willatts et al (2,36,37) used a cloth and barrier so that the object was always invisible, hence their planning tasks required both working memory and planning, as the infant had to remember the toy and where it was placed as well as plan the steps to retrieve it. In the current study, a transparent barrier and box (see figure 1) rather than opaque ones were used so that the goal object was always visible, thus eliminating the contaminating effects of working memory from the task.

3. The selection of goal objects. It has been found from the pilot study that infants are more interested in toys which represent animals and people than other objects. In the current study, graspable toy animals and people were used as goal objects in the planning task.

A description of the subtasks (steps) which comprised the planning task used in the current study is presented below.

Description of the planning task

A sample of the type of materials used in the planning task is shown in Figure 1, followed by a description of the steps of the task (see table 1a).

The 1- to 3-step planning tasks used in the current study were based on those used by Willatts et al (2,36,37).

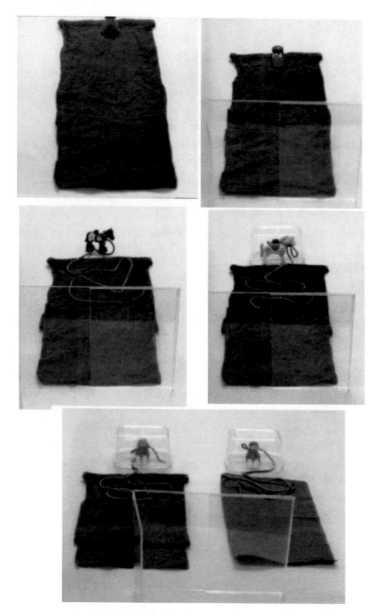

Figure 1. Materials used for the planning tasks.

The 4- and 5-step tasks were added based on the pilot study to avoid the ceiling effect of the task with the 12 month old infants. The 4-step task was designed for the current study and the 5-step task was modified from the work of Chen et al (25).

1. *1-step task.* A cloth was placed on the table in front of the infant. An attractive object (toy) was placed on the cloth such that the child could reach the cloth but could not reach the object. The infant therefore had to pull the cloth in order to retrieve the object.

2. *2-step task.* The cloth and goal object were placed in front of the infant as in the 1-step task; however a transparent barrier was placed between the front of the cloth and the infant so that the infant had to remove the barrier before pulling the cloth to retrieve the object.

3. *3-step task.* The barrier, cloth and goal object were placed in front of the infant as in the 2-step task; however a string was attached to the toy and the string was put on the cloth out of the infant's reach. Thus to attain the toy the infant had to remove the barrier, pull the cloth to bring the string into reach, and then pull the string to get the toy.

4. *4-step task.* The 4-step task was the same as the 3-step task except that the toy was placed inside the Perspex box, so that the child had to remove the barrier, pull the cloth, pull the string, and remove the Perspex box in order to obtain the toy.

5. *5-step task.* In the 5-step task the barrier was placed in front of two cloths on each of which was a string. A toy inside a Perspex box was placed beyond the end of each cloth, but only one string was attached to the toy. To retrieve the toy, the infant needed to remove the barrier, pull the relevant cloth, then pull the relevant string which was attached to the toy to bring the box within reach, and finally remove the Perspex box to obtain the toy. This required the infants to plan in their minds the correct route to the final goal prior to their action.

For the 1-step to 4-step tasks, infants are required to remove or overcome one to four obstacles along the path to the goal. For the 5-step tasks, infants also had to choose between two paths to the goal. They had to see which toy was attached to the string and which one was not in order to decide which cloth to pull.

The goal toys were changed from trial to trial. The inter-trial interval was 20 seconds. During the inter-trial interval, the experimenter gave a toy to the infant to play with while the next trial was prepared.

In the 1-step task a time limit of 30 s was set for each trial starting from the infants' first contact with the cloth to the first contact with the toy.

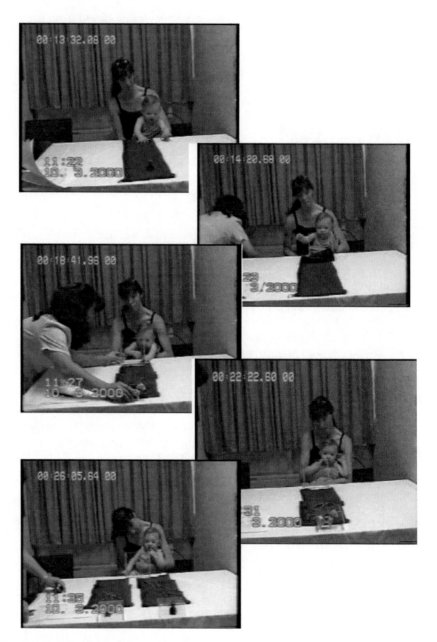

Figure 2.1- to 5-step planning tasks.

On all subsequent trials timing started from first contact with the barrier. A time limit of 30 s was allowed for the 2-step and 3-step tasks, 40 s for the 4-

step task and 50 s for the 5-step task. The time limit for 1-step to 3-step tasks was selected on the basis of findings from Willatts et al.'s (2, 36, 37) studies. The time allowed for the 4-step and 5-step tasks was based on findings from the pilot study.

Table 1a. Steps in the Planning Task

	Objects used	Action required	Time limits for each task (s)
1-step	• Cloth • Toy	1. Pull the cloth to retrieve the toy	30 s
2-step	• Barrier • Cloth • Toy	1. Remove the barrier 2. Pull the cloth to retrieve the toy	30 s
3-step	• Barrier • Cloth • String (attached to toy) • Toy	1. Remove the barrier 2. Pull the cloth 3. Pull the string to retrieve the toy	30 s
4-step	• Barrier • Cloth • String (attached to toy) • Perspex box • Toy (inside Perspex box)	1. Remove the barrier 2. Pull the cloth 3. Pull the string 4. Remove the Perspex box to retrieve the toy	40 s
5 step	• Barrier • Two cloths • Two strings (one of which is attached to a toy) • Two Perspex boxes • Two toys (inside Perspex boxes)	1. Remove the barrier 2. Pull the relevant cloth 3. Pull the relevant string 4. Remove the Perspex box to retrieve the toy	50 s

Criteria for determining ceiling level of performance on the planning task

At each level of the task (i.e., 1-step, 2-step etc.) the task was presented three times. If the child obtained the toy within the time limits on at least one of the three trials at a particular level, testing continued to the next level of the task. If the child failed to obtain the toy for all three trials or the time limit on all three trials at a particular level elapsed, testing was terminated and this was assumed to represent the ceiling of the child's abilities.

Perinatal variables: Medical complications, birthweight and gestation age

It is possible that some factors associated with being preterm affected performance of planning more than prematurity per se. These factors include medical complications, lower birthweight and shorter gestation age. Further analyses were conducted to assess the effect of perinatal variables which might have significantly affected preterm infants' performance on planning measures.For each of these factors the preterm infant group was divided into higher and lower risk groups, and the performance of each of these groups on planning measures was compared to that of the total full term infant group. Birthweight and gestation age were taken as separate factors in the analysis because there were eight preterm infants who were small for gestation age, therefore there was no correlation between birthweight and gestation age. Preterm infants were firstly grouped on the basis of their severity of medical complication:

1. high-risk preterm group ($n = 17$), group 1;
2. low-risk preterm group ($n = 20$), group 2; and,
3. no medical complications (term infants $n = 74$), group 3.

Preterm infants were also grouped on the basis of birthweight:

1. Extremely low birth infant group with birthweight 1000grams or less (n=16), group 1;
2. Very low birth weight infant group with birthweight 1001 to 1500 grams (n=21), group 2;
3. Normal birthweight infant group with birthweight 2501 to 4000gram (n=74), group 3

Finally, Preterm infants were grouped on the basis of gestation age:

1. Shortest gestation age with grestation age less than 28 weeks (n=17), group 1;
2. Short gestatation age with gestation age 28-32 weeks (n=20), group 2;
3. Normal gestation age with gestation age 38-42 weeks (n=74), group 3.

Demographic factors

Infants and their mothers were also assessed on the following confounding factors in the present study: infant motor and mental development, infant temperament, maternal education, family income, maternal psychological well-being.

Procedure

Mothers completed the background information form when the testing session was completed. Assessments for all infants were conducted in a testing room at Mater Children's Hospital. Infants and their mothers were videotaped as they participated in the planning tasks to permit later scoring of these tasks and the calculation of inter-rater reliability scores.

A familiarisation phase preceded testing sessions to enable each infant to become familiar with the experimenter and testing environment. In this phase, the infant was given a toy to play with for about two minutes. The experimenter described the study and gave instructions to the mother while the infant was playing. The mothers were instructed (a) not to give any help or clues to assist their infant's performance on any of the task, (b) to restrain baby's arms or body gently as instructed by the examiner during the delay time between hiding the object and when the infant was allowed to retrieve it in the working memory task, and (c) to ask for a break during the assessment if they felt it was necessary, for example, when the infant was hungry, sleepy, thirsty and so on. The mother was given time to feed the baby and change the infant's nappy before the assessment started.

Instruction of the assessment

The description of the tasks and the instructions given to the mother by the experimenter were found to be appropriate. The instruction given to the infants such as "find the toy" during the infant working memory and planning task gave no clues to the solution and all infants attempted the tasks at the simplest level. On the basis of this evidence no changes were made to the instructions for the study.

The difficulty of the task

Only the 1-step, 2-step and 3-step tasks were originally designed for the planning task, however these produced a ceiling effect and did not demonstrate the full range of the abilities of the 11 month full-term infants. The 4- and 5-step tasks were then designed in the pilot study for the assessment of 10-11 month old infants. It has been found that two full-term infants at 10-11 months could complete the 4-step task, and one of them could complete the 5-step task. Therefore it was decided to add 4- and 5-step tasks in the infant planning tasks.

The determination of time limit

The time limit for the planning tasks from 1-step to 5-step was designed to be 30 s each based on a study by Willatts (2). For the planning task, the time limit which had been set for the 1-step to 3-step tasks was appropriate and no changes were made. However, the time required for the infants to complete the 4- and 5-step tasks was more than 30 s in the current study. It was decided to allow infants to complete the 4-step task in 40 s and the 5-step task in 50 s. The total time for the Infant planning task was about 5 minutes depending upon the performance of the infants. In consideration of the attention span of the infants and the total duration of the testing session which infants were likely to be able to sustain, it was decided to have a break after the assessment of the planning task to avoid fatigue and loss of interest. As the tasks changed regularly and the toys were changed systematically, no difficulty was encountered in maintaining the interest of infants in the tasks.

Toys used in the executive function and sustained attention tasks

A variety of toys was selected for use in the infant planning tasks. The infant's interest in the toys was judged by the infant smiling on seeing the toy, reaching for it, choosing it over other toys, playing with it, or protesting or resisting when the toy was taken away.

Small dolls were used as the goal objects in the 1- and 2-step planning tasks. Animals (such as horses) were used in the 3-step task and different dolls were used in the 4- and 5-step tasks. Three different objects were used for each level of the planning task, and these were changed from trial to trial (see Figure 1).

Findings

Chi-square was used to campare the difference between preterm and full term infants in maternal education, family income, mother's depression level, and infant temperament. One-way Analysis of Variance was used to compare the difference between preterm and full-term infants in Bayley motor and Bayley mental scores. The details of the demographic characteristics is detailed in published articles (33, 34). Preterm infants had significantly lower scores than full-term infants on the assessment about psychomotor development (Bayley PDI). There were no significant differences between the groups for scores on assessment about maternal education, family income, mother's depression level, and infant temperament, and Bayley mental score.

Table 1b indicates that preterm infants had significantly lower score than full-terminfants at both eight month and 10-11 months chronological age in planning tasks from one to five steps between preterm infants and eight month full-term infants.

Table 1b. The Comparison of Preterm and Full-term Infants on Planning Measures at 10-11 Months Chronological Age and eight month corrected age

Planning tasks	Preterm (n=37) P	Full term 8 month (n=74) T1	Full term 10 month (n=68) T2	F	p
One step	1.27(1.79)	2.32(2.05)	3.29(1.98)	12.45***	P<T1* P<T2*** T1<T2*
Two-step	2.84(3.75)	5.59(4.23)	7.53(3.68)	16.57***	P<T1*** P<T2*** T1<T2**
Three-step	4.93(6.00)	9.74(6.71)	12.37(5.89)	16.33***	P<T1*** P<T2*** T1<T2*
Four-step	3.72(7.13)	9.95(9.19)	13.71(8.49)	15.94***	P<T1*** P<T2*** T1<T2*
Five-step	1.24(4.60)	4.32(7.73)	8.61(10.79)	9.85***	P<T2*** T1<T2**
1-5 steps total	17.58(19.78)	36.90(24.81)	49.79(29.55)	18.32***	P<T1** P<T2*** T1<T2*

Note.The values in bold are the means *M* and standard deviations *SD* of transformed data corresponding to the mean of the raw data.

Preterm infants has significantly lower scores than 10-11 month full-term infants in six step task. All 10-11 full-term infants had significant improvement in planning tasks from one-step to six-step tasks, suggesting planning abilities are developing in infants from 8 month to 10-11 month chronological age.

Table 2 demonstrates that Table 2 indicates that preterm infants had significantly longer time required than full-terminfants at both eight month and 10-11 months chronological age in completing planning tasks from one- to six-step planning tasks.

Table 2. The Comparison of Preterm and Full-term Infants on Planning Measures at 10-11 Months Chronological Age and eight month corrected age in completing time in planning tasks

Planning tasks	Preterm (n=37) P	Full term 8 month (n=74) T1	Full term 10 month (n=68) T2	F	p
One step	28.93(23.22)	13.53(11.99)	10.80(7.87)	21.21***	P<T1** P<T2*** T1<T2*
Two-step	48.82(16.08)	31.77(21.73)	23.39(15.99)	21.56***	P<T1** P<T2*** T1<T2*
Three-step	50.72(15.26)	29.01(20.66)	25.50(15.47)	25.45***	P<T1** P<T2*** T1<T2*
Four-step	53.85(13.66)	24.63(22.14)	25.10(18.48)	32.90***	P<T1** P<T2*** T1<T2*
Five-step	57.74(10.49)	14.12(21.78)	21.13(21.89)	61.91***	P<T1** P<T2*** T1<T2*

Note. The values in bold are the means *M* and standard deviations *SD* of transformed data corresponding to the mean of the raw data.

It is possible that some factors associated with being preterm affected performance of planning more than prematurity per se. These factors include medical complications, lower birthweight and shorter gestation age. Further analyses were conducted to assess the effect of perinatal variables which might have significantly affected preterm infants' performance on planning measures.

For each of these factors the preterm infant group was divided into higher and lower risk groups, and the performance of each of these groups on planning measures was compared to that of the total full term infant group.

Birthweight and gestation age were taken as separate factors in the analysis because there were eight preterm infants who were small for gestation age, therefore there was no correlation between birthweight and gestation age. Preterm infants were firstly grouped on the basis of their severity of medical complication:

1. high-risk preterm group ($n = 17$), group 1;
2. low-risk preterm group ($n = 20$), group 2; and,
3. no medical complications (term infants $n = 74$), group 3.

Preterm infants were also grouped on the basis of birthweight:

1. Extremely low birth infant group with birthweight less than 1000grams or less (n=16), group 1;
2. Very low birth weight infant group with birthweight 1000 to 1500 grams (n=21), group 2;
3. Normal birthweight infant group with birthweight 2501 to 4000gram (n=74), group 3

Finally, Preterm infants were grouped on the basis of gestation age:

1. Shortest gestation age with grestation age less than 28 weeks (n=17), group 1;
2. Short gestatation age with gestation age 28-32 weeks (n=20), group 2;
3. Normal gestation age with gestation age 38-42 weeks (n=74), group 3.

The results of the ANOVA for the effect of medical risks on the performance of preterm infants on planning tasks are shown in Table3 along with Tukey's HSD for the pairs of groups.

Discussion

Preterm birth is a common phenomenon which causes the fetus to be exposed to external stimulation whilst many organs are very immature. This provides opportunities to examine factors that may influence the development of a range of abilities.

Table 3. The Comparison of high risk, low risk infants and full-term infants on measures of planning at eight months corrected age

Variables	High-risk preterm infants (n=17)	Low-risk preterm infants (n=20)	Full-term Infants (8ms) (n=74)	Full Term (10ms)	F	p	Tukey's HSD
Birthweight ELBT(n=21) LB(n =16)	14.78 (21.25)	21.25 (23.52)	36.44 (24.65)	49.79 (29.55)	12.46	.00	A <C (.01)** A < D (.00)*** C<D (.05)* B<D(.00)***
Gestration ShorterGA (n=15) LowGA (n=22)	8.1 (10.88)	24.05 (22.00)	36.90 (24.81)	49.79 (29.55)	13.56	.00	A <C (.01)** A < D (.00)*** C<D (.05)* B<D(.00)***
Medical complication Highrisk (n=17) Lowrisk (n=20)	15.38 (20.43)	19.45 (19.54)	36.89 (24.81)	49.79 (29.55)	12.24	.00	A <.C (.01)** A < D (.00)*** B<C (.05)* C<D (.05)* B<D***

Notes.
1. The values in bold are the mean *M* and standard deviation *SD* of
transformed data corresponding to the mean and standard deviations of the raw data. Transformed data were used for the analysis due to the raw data were not normally distributed.
2. HSD: Tukey's Honestly Significant Difference Test. Only Tukey's HSD showing significant differences are reported.

The study reported in this thesis focused specifically on the development planning in infancy, as there has been growing acceptance that these abilities emerge and can be measured during the first year of life (40, 41). These nascent abilities are likely to play a critical role in later cognitive development. For example, there is increasing evidence that deficits in planning underlie learning difficulties observed in school age children (42, 43). As the prevalence of learning problems is very high in preterm infants when they reach school age, there is an increased chance of being able to isolate factors which predispose children to these problems by studying a preterm population.

In the present study, preterm and full-term infants of the same chronological age and same corrected age were compared on measures of planning in order to assess the differential effects of maturation (biological maturity) and length of exposure to extrauterine environmental stimuli on the development of these abilities. Although a number of studies suggest that global development seems to be largely the result of maturational influence (29, 44, 45), others have reported that "neural sculpting" occurs as the result of exposure to environmental influences (46,47). Currently little is known about the impact of the environment on the development of brain mechanisms that mediate specific cognitive abilities, such as planning ability.

The present study found that preterm infants were inferior to full-term infants on planning tasks at both the same chronological age and the same corrected age, but the differences in performance were much less when the infants were compared at the same corrected age. This suggests that maturation had a greater impact than exposure to environmental stimuli on the development of planning. However, as differences between the preterm and full term infants remained even when they were compared on corrected age, other factors must also have impact on the development of planning ability in these infants.

The study found that preterm infants who had high medical risk in the perinatal period performed worse than those who did not have these medical risk factors on measures planning, although the differences in performance were not statistically significant. The scores of the preterm infant groups were in the high risk group were lower than those of full-term infants on planning measures. These differences reached statistical significance between preterm infants and full-term infants, and additionally between the low medical raks preterm group and the full-term infants at eight month corrected age. The difference between preterm infants who had high medical risk and full-term infants was greater than that between low-risk infants and full-term infants on planning measures, suggesting that medical risk influences the development of planning ability.

ELBW was defined as birthweight < 1,000 g. Preterm infants in the < 1000 g birthweight group did not differ from the preterm infants with > 1000 g birthweight group with regards to medical risk status. Two gestation age groups comprised infants with gestation age < 28 weeks and preterm infants with > 28 weeks gestation age. Infants with gestation age < 28 weeks were regarded as having shorter gestation age. Likewise, preterm infants born at < 28 weeks gestation were not significantly different to those with 28-32 weeks gestation in terms of medical risk status. There was therefore an opportunity to consider the effect of birthweight and gestation age independent of medical complications. In each case, the high-risk group (i.e., the <1000 g birthweight group, and the < 28 weeks gestation group) performed more poorly than their low risk counterparts (i.e., the > 1000 g birthweight group, and the > 28 weeks gestation group) on planning measures although these differences did not reach statistical significance. The performance of the high risk on measures of planning were also consistently poorer than that of the full-term group, and this reached levels of statistical significance. The performance of the low risk group on measures of planning were poorer than that of the full-term group in 10-11 chronologial age. These findings suggest that medical risk, lower birthweight, and lower gestation age more adversely affect performance on the planning measures in addition to premature birh per se. The difference between low risk preterm infant groups is more frequent than that of the full-term infants between eight months and 10-11 months chronolgical age suggesting prematury birth had also adversely affect performance on the planning measure in risk risk preterm infants.

Findings in the present study are consistent with those of other researchers, who have reported that perinatal risk factors influence cognitive development during the first year of life (48-50). Ross et al. (50) for example reported high risk preterm infants showed lower scores on measures of working memory during infancy, but they did not examine planning which have been found in the present study. Similar deficits in EF have also been reported in studies of school age children who were born preterm and who experienced high medical risk (31,51). For example, Luciana et al. (31) found that preterm born children at 7 to 9 years of age who had high medical risk differed from full-term infants on executive function tasks, and Taylor, Klein, et al (52) also suggested that medical risk may influence the long term developmental outcomes of preterm infants.

The findings in the present study are also consistent with previous studies of children with extremely low birthweight, whether defined as birthweight < 1,000 g (53) or < 750 g (51), which have reported lower scores on the performance of planning tasks. However the children in these studies were older than the children in the present study. The effect of SGA may also influence the performance of planning in the preterm infants with < 1000 g birthweight group in the current study. For example, the poorer performance of the ELBW infants on EF may have been due to the fact that there were eight

SGA infants in the ELBW group. Several studies, such as that of McCarton et al. (54) have reported that SGA preterm infants tend to perform more poorly than their AGA counterparts on general developmental assessment measures. In the current study, SGA preterm infants tend to show poorer scores on the planning measures than AGA preterm infants, but these differences did not reach statistically significant differences as the number of SGA infants in the present study was too small. Evidence for direct central nervous system effects of intrauterine undernutrition is primarily based on animal studies.

In the present study, both preterm infants with < 28 weeks gestation and infants with 28-32 weeks gestation had lower scores than the full-term infants on planning measures. The differences between high risk preterm groups and full-term infants reached statistical significance on measures planning. This suggests that a shorter gestation age is detrimental to performance in planning.

There is considerable evidence that tasks which require planning a sequence of steps are regulated by the dorsolateral prefrontal cortex (16,17). The deficits in measures of planning observed in the high perinatal risk groups may be associated with the adverse effects of these perinatal risk factors on the prefrontal cortex which is very immature and sensitive in the preterm infants (55-57). Mouradian, Als, and Coster (58) suggested that deficits in planning might be due to late maturing cortical organization, particularly of the prefrontal regions. Myelination of the brain has been demonstrated to occur in a systematic fashion starting at the end of the first trimester and continuing at least until the end of the second year (59). Between 23 and 32 weeks of gestation, structural differentiation of the central nervous system is at its most rapid (i.e., neuronal differentiation, glial cell growth, myelination, axonal and dendritic growth and synapse formation). The preterm infants in the present study were born between 24 to 32 weeks gestation just at this time of brain development. Most of these preterm infants were in the NICU for up to three months after they were born. The environment in the NICU may not be conductive to the development of the brain and the perinatal risk factors which occurred during this period may have further adversely affect brain development. The prefrontal cortex, which appears to play a central role in regulating planning, is a late maturing area of the brain, and is consequently likely to be particularly vulnerable to damage in preterm infants (60). Those preterm infants with these detrimental perinatal events are at particular risk for the abnormal prefrontal cortex functioning, hence the deficits in planning.

The deficits of planning observed in preterm infants may have long term consequences in terms of learning difficulties at school age. During school years, children born preterm who experienced high perinatal risks (i.e., high medical risks, extremely low birthweight, shorter gestation age) during the perinatal period have been found to have higher rates of deficits in cognitive and neuropsychological abilities, mathematics achievement, and adaptive behaviours, as well as higher rates of special education placements as compared with their full-term counterparts (31,52,61,62). It is possible that this is due to early abnormality in the development of the prefrontal cortex and consequent executive dysfunction. Anderson et al (63) suggested that this might possibly result in inability to ever acquire aspects of EF.

Both low risk and high-risk preterm infant groups differed significantly from full-term infants on SA measures. This may be attributable to their early physical environment. In the NICU where most preterm infants spent the first 2-3 months of their lives, they were typically over-stimulated with high levels of light, sound and multiple painful procedures. They also experienced maternal separation for prolonged periods. Gardner and Karmel (64) suggested that these adverse environmental conditions during the perinatal period may be associated with a lowered functional and structural coherence or integrity within the central nervous system and hence poor attentional skills. Experimental evidence from animal models has further shown that these adverse environmental factors in the perinatal period may lead to neuronal cell death in the immature brain (65). An EEG study on children who had attentional deficits found that these children showed excessively slow activity and decreased alpha power in the left and right hemisphere across the frontal, parietal, and temporal brain regions when they performed the Continuous Performance Task. This suggests that they may have had a state of low central nervous system cortical arousal due to dysfunction in the subcortical centers (66). Volumetric measurement of brain regions in 8-years-old children born preterm showed disproportionately smaller volumes of the anterior cortical areas which are associated with increased incidence of attentional deficits and other behavioural disorders (67). Biological and environmental insults associated with preterm birth may have resulted in differences in the architecture of these regions in preterm infants compared to typically developing full-term infants.

In summary, psychomotor development as measured by the PDI on the Bayley Scales of Infant Development significantly contributed to the differences between preterm and full-term infants' scores planning. Infant temperament and maternal psychological and socio-economic factor had little effect on planning. Medical risk factors, extremely low birthweight, and shorter gestation age confounded the effects of prematurity for planning measures.

Conclusion

Two major conclusions can be drawn from the present studies.Differences were found between preterm and full-term infants on measures of planning at both the same corrected and same chronological age. Maturation was found to be an important factor influencing the development of planning. However other factors associated with prematurity were also found to affect performance on measures of planning.

The present research examined the factors which may significantly affect the differences between preterm and full-term infants. In particular, high medical risk, lower birthweight, and shorter gestation age all affected the differences between preterm and full-term infants on measures of planning.

Limitation

The limitation for the present study is that the coding scheme for the planning task, which was based on that used by Willatts et al. (2, 36, 37) is very conservative and only infants who fixated on the goal and retrieved the toy were judged to be full intentional. As no partial scores were permitted and few preterm infants met these rigid criteria when the tasks had more than two steps, the range of scores for the preterm infants was quite restricted. Another limitation of the study due to the restricted timeframe is that long-term outcomes cannot be assessed. Hence a link cannot be made to the preterm infants between the deficits in EF and SA found in the present study and learning difficulties in school. Finally, it must be emphasised that inferences about the relation between performance on planning and the development of dorsalateral regions of the prefrontal cortex, and also inferences about the effects of perinatal risk factors on the development of the prefrontal cortex are speculative, and based on behavioural observations as no direct measures of either the structure or functioning of the brain using neuro-imaging techniques was possible for such young infants.

Implications

The fact that the present study has demonstrated that planning can be measured relatively easily in infants should lead to the development and standardisation of an assessment tool which can be used to assess the development of these specific cognitive skills during infancy. Ideally such a tool should refine the tests used in the present study, with special attention to the development of techniques which will allow the assessment of planning. Such an assessment tool may prove to be more useful than the currently available measures of overall development for predicting later learning outcomes. The results of the study draw attention to the fact that even infants who have no obvious neurological abnormalities, and whose general development is within the average range, may nevertheless have problems in specific areas of cognitive development. This suggests that these specific cognitive abilities should be routinely assessed in the follow-up of high-risk infants. Further research will however be needed to assess the accuracy of such assessments in identifying infants who subsequently experience learning difficulties and attention deficits.

References

[1]   Bhutta AT, Cleves MA, Casey PH, Cradock MM, Anand KJS. Cognitive and behavioral outcomes of school-aged children who were born preterm: A meta-analysis. JAMA 2002;288(6):728-37.

[2]   Willatts P. Development of means-end behavior in young infants: Pulling a support to retrieve a distant object. Dev Psychol 1999;35(3):651-67.

[3]   Willatts P. Beyond the "Couch Potato" infant: How infants use their knowledge to regulate action, solve problems, and achieve goals. In: Bremner G, Slater A, Butterworth G, eds. Infant development: Recent advances. Hove, East Sussex: Psychology Press, 1997:109-35.

[4]   Bauer PJ, Schwade JA, Wewerka SS, Delaney K. Planning ahead: Goal-directed problem solving by 2-year-olds. Dev Psychol 1999;35(5):1321-37.

[5]   Olson CR, Gettner SN. Representation of object-centered space in the primate frontal lobe. In: Ito M, editor. Brain and mind: For better understanding of the dynamic function of mind and its supporting brain mechanism. Amsterdam: Elsevier Science, 1997:275-93.

[6]   Willatts P, Rosie K. Thinking ahead: Development of means-end planning in young infants. Infant Behav Dev 1992;15:769.

[7]   Friedman SL, Scholnick EK. An evolving "Blueprint" for planning: Psychological requirements, task characteristics, and social-cultural influences. In: Friedman SL, Scholnick EK, editors. The developmental psychology of planning: Why, how, and when do we plan? Mahwah, NJ: Lawrence Erlbaum, 1997:3-22.

[8]   Bishop DVM, Aamodt-Leeper G, Creswell C, McGurk CR, Skuse DH. Individual differences in cognitive planning on the Tower of Hanoi task: Neuropsychological maturity or measurement error? J Child Psychol Psychiatry 2001;42(4):551-6.

[9] Haith MM. The development of future thinking as essential for the emmergence of skill in planning. In: Friedman SL, Scholnick EK, eds. The developmental psychology of planning: Why, how and when do we plan? Mahwah, NJ: Lawrence Erlbaum, 1997:25-42.

[10] Willatts P. Development of problem-solving strategies in infancy. In: Bjorklund DF, editor. Children's strategies: Contemporary views of cognitive development. Hillsdale, NJ: Lawrence Erlbaum, 1990:23-66.

[11] Scholnick EK, Friedman SL. Planning in context: Developmental and situational considerations. Int J Behav Dev 1993;16(2):145-67.

[12] Borys SV, Spitz HH, Dorans BA. Tower of Hanoi performance of retarded young adults and nonretarded children as a function of solution length and goal state. J Exp Child Psychol 1982;33:87-110.

[13] Luria AR. The working brain. New York: Basic Books; 1973.

[14] Shallice T, Burgess PW. Deficits in strategy application following frontal lobe damage in man. Brain 1991;114:727-41.

[15] Ozonoff S, Pennington BF, Rogers SJ. Executive function deficits in high-functioning autistic individuals: Relationship to theory of mind. J Child Psychol Psychiatry 1991;32(7):1081-105.

[16] Levin HS, Song J, Ewing-Cobbs L, Roberson G. Porteus Maze performance following traumatic brain injury in children. Neuropsychology 2001;15(4):557-67.

[17] Morris RG, Miotto EC, Feigenbaum JD, Bullock P, Polkey CE. Planning ability after frontal and temporal lobe lesions in humans: The effects of selection equivocation and working memory load. Cogn Neuropsychol 1997;14(7):1007-27.

[18] Scheibel RS, Levin HS. Frontal lobe dysfunction following closed head injury in children: Findings from neuropsychology and brain imaging. In: Krasnegor NA, Lyon GR, Goldman-Rakic PS, editors. Development of the prefrontal cortex: Evolution, neurobiology, and behavior. Baltimore: Paul H. Brookes, 1997:241-63.

[19] Benton A. Prefrontal injury and behavior in children. Dev Neuropsychol 1991;7(3):275-81.

[20] Goel V, Grafman J. Role of the right prefrontal cortex in ill-structured planning. Cogn Neuropsychol 2000;17(5):415-36.

[21] Graham S, Harris KR. Addressing problems in attention, memory, and executive functioning. In: Lyon GR, Krasnegor NA, editors. Attention, memory, and executive function. Baltimore: Paul H. Brookes, 1996:349-65.

[22] Luria AR. Higher cortical functions in man. New York: Basic Books, 1980.

[23] Milner B, Petrides M. Behavioural effects of frontal-lobe lesions in man. Trends Neurosci 1984;7:403-7.

[24] Walsh KW. Neuropsychology: A clinical approach. Edinburgh: Churchill Livingstone, 1978.

[25] Chen Z, Sanchez RP, Campbell T. From beyond to within their grasp: The rudiments of analogical problem solving in 10- and 13-month-olds. Dev Psychol 1997;33(5):790-801.

[26] Passler MA, Isaac W, Hynd GW. Neuropsychological development of behavior attributed to frontal lobe functioning in children. Dev Neuropsychol 1985;1(4):349-70.

[27] Welsh MC, Pennington BF, Groisser DB. A normative-developmental study of executive function: A window on prefrontal function in children. Dev Neuropsychol 1991;7(2):131-49.

[28] Ross G, Lipper E, Auld PAM. Cognitive abilities and early precursors of learning disabilities in very-low-birthweight children with normal intelligence and normal neurological status. Int J Behav Dev 1996;19(3):563-80.

[29] Rutter M. Developing minds: Challenge and continuity across the life span. London: Penguin, 1992.

[30] McCall RB. What process mediates predictions of childhood IQ from infant habituation and recognition memory? Speculations on the roles of inhibition and rate of information processing. Intelligence 1994;18:107-25.

[31] Luciana M, Lindeke L, Georgieff M, Mills M, Nelson CA. Neurobehavioral evidence for working-memory deficits in school-aged children with histories of prematurity. Dev Med Child Neurol 1999;41:521-33.

[32] Hooper SR, Swartz CW, Wakely MB, de Kruif REL, Montgomery JW. Executive functions in elementary school children with and without problems in written expression. J Learn Disabil 2002;35(1):57-68.

[33] Sun J, Buys N. Prefrontal lobe functioning and its relationship to working memory in preterm infants. Int J Child Adolesc Health 2011;4(1):13-7.

[34] Sun J, Mohay H, O'Callaghan M. Executive function in preterm and full-term infants. Early Hum Dev 2009;85(4):225-30.

[35] Willatts P, Rosie K, editors. Planning by 12-month-old infants. Annual Conference of the Society for Research in Child Development; 1989 April; Kansas City, MO.

[36] Willatts P, Forsyth JS, DiModugno MK, Varma S, Colvin M. Influence of long-chain polyunsaturated fatty acids on infant cognitive function. Lipids 1998;33(10):973-80.

[37] Willatts P, Forsyth JS, DiModugno MK, Varma S, Colvin M. Effect of long-chain polyunsaturated fatty acids in infant formula on problem solving at 10 months of age. Lancet 1998;352:688-91.

[38] Willatts P, ed. Development of means-end planning in the second year of life. International Conference on Infant Studies, Atlanta, GA, 1998.

[39] Willatts P. The infant planning task. Dundee, Scotland: Willatts, 1998.

[40] Diamond A, Doar B. The performance of human infants on a measure of frontal cortex function, the delayed response task. Dev Psychobiol 1989;22(3):271-94.

[41] Diamond A, Gilbert J. Development as progressive inhibitory control of action: Retrieval of a contiguous object. Cogn Dev 1989;4:223-49.

[42] Barkley RA. Behavioral inhibition, sustained attention, and executive functions: Constructing a unifying theory of ADHD. Psychol Bull 1997;121(1):65-94.

[43] Gathercole SE, Pickering SJ. Working memory deficits in children with low achievements in the national curriculum at 7 years of age. Br J Dev Psychol 2000;70:177-94.

[44] Hunt JV, Rhodes L. Mental development of preterm infants during the first year. Child Dev 1977;48:204-10.

[45] Ungerer JA, Sigman M. Developmental lags in preterm infants from one to three years of age. Child Dev 1983;54:1217-28.

[46] Campos JJ, Kermoian R, Witherington D, Chen H, Dong Q. Activity, attention and developmental transitions in infancy. In: Lang PJ, Simons RF, editors. Attention and orienting: Sensory and motivational processes. Mahwah, NJ: Lawrence Erlbaum, 1997:393-415.

[47] Dawson G, Frey K, Panagiotides H, Yamada E, Hessel D, Osterling J. Infants of depressed mothers exhibit atypical frontal electrical brain activity during interactions with mothers and with a familiar nondepressed adult. Child Dev 1999;70:1058-66.

[48] Molfese V, Thomson B. Optimality versus complications: Assessing predictive values of perinatal scales. Child Dev 1985;56:810-23.

[49] Piper MC, Kunos I, Willis DM, Mazer B. Effect of gestational age on neurological functioning of the very low-birthweight infant at 40 weeks. Dev Med Child Neurol 1985;27:596-605.

[50] Ross G, Tesman J, Auld PM, Nass R. Effects of subependymal and mild intraventricular lesions on visual attention and memory in premature infants. Dev Psychol 1992;28(6):1067-74.

[51] Taylor HG, Klein N, Minich NM, Hack M. Middle-school-age outcomes in children with very low birthweight. Child Dev 2000;71:1495-511.

[52] Taylor HG, Klein N, Schatschneider C, Hack M. Predictors of early school age outcomes in very low birth weight children. Dev Behav Pediatr 1998;19(4):235-43.

[53] Harvey JM, O'Callaghan MJ, Mohay H. Executive function of children with extremely low birthweight: A case control study. Dev Med Child Neurol 1999;41:292-7.

[54] McCarton CM, Wallace IF, Divon M, Vaughan HG. Cognitive and neurologic development of the premature, small for gestational age infant through age 6: Comparison by birth weight and gestational age. Pediatrics 1996;98(6):1167-78.

[55] Aylward GP. Perinatal asphyxia: Effects of biological and environmental risks. Clin Perinat 1993;20:433-49.

[56] Diamond A, Lee E. Inability of five-month-old infants to retrieve a contiguous object: A failure of conceptual understanding or of control of action? Child Dev 2000;71(6):1477-94.

[57] Fletcher JM, Brookshire BL, Landry SH, Bohan TP, Davidson KC, Francis DJ, et al. Attentional skills and executive functions in children with early hydrocephalus. Dev Neuropsychol 1996;12(1):53-76.

[58] Mouradian LE, Als H, Coster WJ. Neurobehavioral functioning of healthy preterm infants of varying gestational ages. Dev Behav Pediatr 2000;21(6):408-16.

[59] Battin MR, Maalouf EF, Counsell SJ, Herlihy AH, Rutherford MA, Azzopardi D, et al. Magnetic resonance imaging of the brain in very preterm infants: Visualization of the germinal matrix, early myelination, and cortical folding. Pediatrics 1998;101(6):957-62.

[60] Gilles FH, Shankle W, Dooling EC. Myelinated tracts: Growth pattern. In: Gilles FH, Leviton AD, Dooking EC, editors. The developing human brain: Growth and epidemiologic neuropathology. Baltimore: Williams Wilkins, 1983.

[61] Taylor HG, Anselmo M, Foreman AL, Schatschneider C, Angelopoulos J. Utility of kindergarten teacher judgments in identifying early learning problems. J Learn Disabil 2000;33(2):200-10.

[62] Hack M, Friedman H, Fanaroff AA. Outcomes of extremely low birth weight infants. Pediatrics 1996;98(5):931-7.

[63] Anderson SW, Damasio H, Tranel D, Damasio AR. Long-term sequelae of prefrontal cortex damage acquired in early childhood. Dev Neuropsychol 2000;18(3):281-90.

[64] Gardner JM, Karmel BZ. Attention and arousal in preterm and full-term neonates. In: Field T, Sostek A, editors. Infants born at risk. Boston, MA: Allyn Bacon, 1983: 69-98.

[65] Bhutta AT, Anand KJS. Abnormal cognition and behavior in preterm neonates linked to smaller brain volumes. Trends Neurosci 2001;24:129-32.

[66] El-Sayed E, Larsson J, Persson HE, Rydelius P. Altered cortical activity in children with attention-deficit/hyperactivity disorder during attentional load task. J Am Acad Child Adolesc Psychiatry 2002;41(7):811-9.

[67] Peterson BS, Vohr BR, Staib LH, Cannistraci D, Schneider KC, Katz KH, et al. Regional brain volume abnormalities and long term cognitive outcome in preterm infants. JAMA 2000;284:1939-47.

Chapter V

A comparison of sustained attention in very preterm and term infants

Abstract

This chapter investigates sustained attention in preterm and full-term infants at 8 months after expectd date of delivery. Sustaind attention emerges in infancy and continues to develop throughout childhood. Sustained attention is believed to underlie some learning problems in children at school age. This study investigated sustained attention in preterm and full-term infants at 8 months after expected date of delivery. Thirty-seven preterm infants without identified disabilities, and 74 due date and gender matched healthy full-term infants, participated in the present study. The preterm infants were all less than 32 weeks gestation and less than 1,500 grams birthweight. All infants were therefore assessed on sustained attention tasks at 8 months after the expected date of delivery (when preterm infants were actually 10-11 months chronological age).

The findings of the study showed that preterm infants performed significantly more poorly than full-term infants at both 8 months corrected age and 10-11 month chronological age on measures of sustained attention. Medical risk, lower birthweight and lower gestation age were found not affect the performance on sustained attention tasks. The findings of this study suggests that the deficits of sustained attention in preterm infants may be associated with birth prematurity per se, and that additional complications may not have any further detrimental effect.

Introduction

Advances in medical technologies have led to considerable improvements in the management of premature infants, and resulted in the increased survival of infants of progressively lower birthweight and shorter gestation. Compared with full-term infants, those born early are at increased risk of subsequent developmental difficulties, in both the cognitive, social and emotional, and behavioural domains (1-3). The risk of these adverse outcomes increases as gestation age and birthweight decrease (4).

Sustained attention (SA) has been linked with learning difficulty and attentional deficits in school aged children born preterm (5,6), all of which are more prevalent in children born preterm. SA is effortful and conscious and is associated with cognitive abilities that require exploratory manipulation. Exploration in infants is effortful and related to learning (7). SA refers to the "capacity to maintain focus and alertness over time" (8) and is sometimes referred to as attention span, vigilance, or persistence of effort (9). The dimension of SA was found consistently in factor analytic studies using a battery of neuropsychological tests presumed to assess SA (8,10).

Sergeant (11) described SA as "a skill of maintaining controlled processing performance over time." In this cognitive model, SA is viewed as essential to executive function. Attention plays a role in scrutinising information in the executive control of novel behaviour. That is, certain items of information must be actively attended to, and others must be actively ignored when subjects are required to adapt their behaviour to new situations. Attention is viewed as an active process with a dynamic "management function" that plays an essential role in determining what is selected and sustained for attention. Sergeant points out that this management function is related to what neuropsychologists often refer to as executive function, which is presumed to be regulated by the frontal lobe.

The neuropsychological model on the other hand defines SA as it relates to the concept of vigilance or the ability to maintain performance over extended periods (12). Mirskyet al (8) defined SA as the ability to focus attention not only over a long period of time while responding rapidly to target stimuli, but also inhibiting responses to distractor and other stimuli, such as the Continuous Performance Task (13).

In both the cognitive and neuropsychological models, SA appears to overlap with EF. However, attention is not identical to EF and deserves recognition as a separate, semi-independent component, as the regions in the brain that are involved in the regulation of attention not only include frontal cortex but also involve other regions.

Learning difficulty and attentional deficits are more common in school aged children born preterm than in those born at term (5,6) with those preterm children who had medical complications in the perinatal period being more impaired on SA measures than other preterm children (14).

SA has been assessed in infancy using behavioural indicators, such as maintaining visual examination of an object while simultaneously fingering it, turning it around, and transferring it from hand to hand, which distinguishes it from other less focused attention. One measure of SA is the amount of time infants spend on a task (15).

From 5 to 12 months of age, infants start to demonstrate SA by actively exploring objects in a variety of ways. They use reaching, grasping, and looking. They may also mouth the object, finger it, bang it, push it around, drop or throw it. Developmental changes in exploratory behaviour have been observed between 5 and 12 months of age (16). At 5-7 months infants use mouthing to explore the object. Gradually, as the infant gets older, mouthing recedes and is replaced by more visual-motor actions, such as banging, fingering, and transferring while simultaneously looking. These exploratory behaviours have been found to be important for infant's learning (17).

Non-exploratory behaviour refers to activities which are repetitive and unfocused (e.g., repetitive and stereotyped banging, mouthing or tactile manipulation without visual exploration, or causal glancing without changes in facial expression or tactile manipulation). A measure of non-exploratory behaviour or inattention is the number of off-task glances or brief distractions that interrupt the flow of infant engagement with the object (18,19). Off-task glances have been defined as any situation where infants avert their gaze from the task, accompanied by a temporary cessation of active manipulation such as fingering, rotating, transferring, and mouthing.

Factors such as general development, infant temperament, maternal education, family income, and maternal psychological wellbeing, which could influence infant development and hence performance on the test items, were examined.

The influences of perinatal risk factors including medical complications, lower birthweight, and lower gestation age that may affect infants' performances on SA tasks at eight months after expected date of delivery were also examined. These perinatal variables were used to divide the preterm infants into high-risk and low-risk groups. The performance of these two groups was compared to each other and to that of full-term infants, to provide an indication of the effects of adverse medical factors on the development of SA.

Duration of attention and off-task glances were recoded for infants performance on each task. It was hypothesised that differences on measures of SA would exist between the preterm and full-term infants group even when the influence of confounding variables were taken into account. If this is the case these measures of specific cognitive abilities, which are associated with behaviour and learning, may provide a means of identifying children at risk of school difficulties in infancy. The aims of this study were to compare the difference between preterm and full-term infants in SA. In addition, the relationship between SA and executive function will be examined.

This study was undertaken to compare the performance of preterm and full-term infants of the same corrected age (8 months) age and 10-11 month chronological age on tests related to working memory. Specifically the study tested two hypotheses:

- *Hypothesis 1*: There will be significant difference between preterm and full-term infants of the same chronological age in the performance of sustained attention task (i.e., exposure to extrauterine environmental stimuli is the key factor influencing the development of sustained attention).
- *Hypothesis 2:* There will be significant difference between preterm and full-term infants of the same corrected age in the performance of sustained attention task (i.e., maturation of the central nervous system from the time of conception is the key factors influencing the development of sustained attention).

Our study

All subjects were recruited through the Mater Children's Hospital, Brisbane where they were all born. Both preterm and full-term infants were healthy and without any. There were 37 preterm infants with birthweights of < 1500 g and < 28 weeks gestation and 74 full-term infants with normal birhtweight and gestational age and no medical complications in the perinatal period participated in the study. Full-term infants were matched to preterm infants in age and gender. The purpose of having two full-term comparison groups is to increase the statistical power. All infants were assessed on the attention tasks described below. These measures formed the dependent variables. All infants were tested at eight months (+ or - 2 weeks) after the expected date of delivery. All subjects lived within a 50-kilometre radius of the Mater Mothers' Hospital and were health and free from disabilities at the time of assessment. If they were found to have disabilities, such as developmental delay as measured by the Bayley Scales of Infant Development (i.e., Bayley MDI and PDI scores less than 70), they were excluded from the study. Two full-term infants were excluded from the study.

Participation in the project was voluntary and informed consent was obtained from at least one parent of each child. Ethical approval for the project was obtained from the Mater Children's and Mater Mothers' Hospital Ethics Committees, and the Queensland University of Technology Research Ethics Committee.

Infants and their mothers were also assessed on the following confounding factors in the present study: infant motor and mental development, infant temperament, maternal education, family income, maternal psychological well-being, and perinatal variables (medical complications, birthweight, and gestational age). All infants were assessed on the above variables at 8 months after the expected date of delivery (preterm infants were 10 to 11 months chronological age at this time). The characteristics of the participants can be found in the published paper (20).

Selection of sustained attention measures

SA was assessed using Ruff's (21) Object Examination task. This measure was used as a means of assessing the duration of various forms of exploration of a set of novel objects. This provided a measure of focused (sustained) attention. Five objects which were all graspable and varied in colour, texture, shape and size, were offered to the infant one at a time in a fixed order for one minute each. For eight-month-old infants the objects were a puzzle, chain, phone, squeezable rubber rabbit, and a wooden bell (Figure 1). These toys were selected based on a pilot study, which found that most infants showed an interest in them and that eight-month-old infants could handle and manipulate them.

From the five one-minute sessions, two measures of SA were calculated.

1. Duration of SA. This reflects the persistence of effort by the infant. An episode of SA was identified when the infant leaned in towards

and fixated on an object while simultaneously manipulating it, fingering it, turning it around, transferring it from hand to hand, slowly banging it against a table, or mouthing it and looking at it immediately afterwards (22). The end of a period of SA was recorded when the infant looked away and/or stopped actively engaging with the object (e.g., when repetitive and non-focused activity occurred, such as banging the object in a rapid, repetitive way without looking at it, mouthing the object without looking at it afterwards, or fingering, rotating or transferring the object from hand to hand without looking at it).

2. Number of off-task glances. An off-task glance marked the end of an attention episode and the look back marked the onset of a new episode. Off-task glances were defined as any look away from the task, accompanied by a temporary cessation of active exploration. This measure quantified brief distractions that seemed to interrupt the flow of infant engagement.

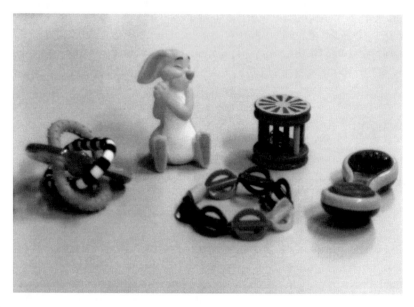

Figure 1.Toys for infant sustained attention task at 8 months.

Videotapes of the SA task were coded using the *Observer* software for collection and analysis of observational data (23). The *Observer* software generated the descriptive statistics (frequency and duration) indicating SA, such as looking at the object while fingering, rotating, transferring from hand to hand, banging slowly or mouthing followed by immediately looking at it, across the five toys for the duration of attention and off-task glances.

A description of the SA task and the variables of SA used in this study are presented in Table 1.

Table 1. Summary of sustained attention task

Task	Behaviour indicating SA	Duration of off-task glances:	Duration of the episode of SA
Five objects, varying in colour, texture, shape, and size, presented one at a time, for one minute. (i.e., total time 5 minute)	Looking at object while fingering, rotating, transferring from hand to hand, banging slowly or mouthing followed by immediately looking at it.	Looking away from the object, and ceasing to engage the object	From the onset of exploration of the object, until the infant looks away from the object when there is off task glance.
Scoring		Average duration of off-task on 5 objects was calculated to indicate the duration of off-task glances	Average duration of exploration was calculated for five 1-minute object examinations.

Confounding factors

The Bayley Scales of Infant Development (BS1D II) (24) were used to provide a standard measure of infant development. The mental development scale includes items that assess memory, habituation, vocalization, language and social skills and the psychomotor development scale assesses the ability to control the gross and fine muscle groups. A mean and standard deviation for Mental Development Index (MDI) and Psychomotor Development Index (PDI) are 100 and 15 respectively.

The Australian revised version of the Infant Temperament Questionnaire (25) was used to assess infant temperament. This is a 30-item questionnaire on which parents rate various aspects of the child's behaviour on a six-point rating scale from almost never (score 1) to almost always (score 6). Infant temperament was classified as easy, average, or difficult based on the norms for Australian children provided by Sanson et al (31).

Maternal psychological wellbeing was measured by the General Health Questionnaire (GHQ) (26), which provides a measure of maternal symptoms of anxiety and depression. Mothers scoring 13 or more were regarded as having signs of anxiety and depression whilst those with lower scores were regarded as having normal psychological status.

Maternal education and family income, were recorded from the demographic information sheet completed by parents. Infant perinatal information was obtained from medical records at the Mater Mother's hospital. These included birth weight, gestational age, interuterine growth retardation, and the following medical complications; home oxygen dependency (HOME O2), [defined as continuing to need supplemental oxygen at home following hospital discharge] ventricular dilatation (VD), periventricular leukomalacia (PVL), and cerebro-ventricular haemorrhage (CVH). For the purpose of this study a "high medical risk" very preterm infant was defined as a very preterm infant who had one or more of these medical complications.

Procedure for the assessment

Infants were tested individually. All assessments were conducted in a quiet testing room located in the Department of Child Health at the Mater Children's Hospital, Brisbane. Infants sat on their mother's lap adjacent to one side of the testing table and facing the video camera. The table was rectangular (90cm×75cm) and covered with a white sheet. The examiner sat at 90 degrees to the infant so as not to obscure the view of the video camera.

Infants and their mothers were videotaped during the SA tasks for the purpose of scoring and for rating inter-rater reliability. A familiarisation phase included infants getting used to the testing environment, and instructing mothers not to help with the testing. Following this, the experimenter played with the child for a few minutes using toys which were not to be used for the testing.

The sequence in which the tasks were presented was: SA task, and Bayley Scales of Infant Development. Following these assessments, all mothers were asked to complete the demographic information questionnaire, GHQ, and Infant Temperament Questionnaire.

The first author scored all SA tasks. Another coder who had a background in developmental psychology scored 10 percent of the infants tested at eight months corrected age. Agreement for the trials with SA was 95%.

Very preterm infants had significantly lower scores than full-term infants on the psychomotor development scale (PDI) of the BSID II but no significant differences were found between the groups on the mental development scale (MDI) or any of the other variables (see table 2). Bayley PDI were entered as a covariate in an analysis of co-variance (ANCOVA) model (adjusted model) to examine their effect on the differences between very preterm and full-term infants on SA measures (see Table 3).

Table 2. Comparison of very preterm and full-term infants on infant and maternal variables

Variables	Preterm (n = 37)	Full-term (n = 74)	t or χ2	*p*
Bayley MDI M*(SD)*	111.6 (5.6)	110.9 (6.6)	t = 0.53	0.59
Bayley PDI M*(SD)*	97.5 (13.1)	106.8 (8.3)	t= 4.55	**0.00**
Temperament Easy n (%) Average n (%) Difficult n (%)	20 (54.1) 11 (29.7) 6 (16.2)	43 (58.1) 18 (24.3) 13 (17.6)	χ2 = .94	0.9
Maternal education n(%) ≤Grade 12 n(%) >Grade 12	26 (78.8) 7 (21.2)	48(64.9) 26(35.1)	χ2 = 2.1	0.2
Family income p.a. n(%) 30,000 and less n(%) 30,001-59,999 n(%) 60,000 and above	13 (35.1) 19 (51.4] 5(13.5)	16(21.6) 41(55.4) 17(23.0)	χ2= 0.2	0.2
Maternal Psychological wellbeing (GHQ scores) n(%)score ≤ 12 n(%) score >12	32 (86.5) 5(13.5)	66(89.2) 8(10.8)	χ2= 2.4	0.3

What we found

Table 3 shows the results of a MANOVA used to examine group differences in the performance of SA tasks by preterm and full-term infants at eight month corrected age. The univariate ANOVAs show that there were significant differences between the groups on both components of SA at eight month corrected age and 10-11 month chronological age, as the scores of the preterm infants remained below those of the term infants. It is therefore important to examine whether this difference was due to confounding variables or whether it was due to prematurity per se.

Table 3. The Comparison of Preterm and Full-term Infants on Sustained Attention Measures at 10-11 Months Chronological Age and eight month corrected age

	Sustained attention	Preterm (n=37)	Full term (n=74)	F	p
Comparison at 10-11 month chronological age	1.Duration of attention M (SD)	11.40 (9.90) **2.19 (.65)**	51.75 (10.74) **8.24 (2.82)**	69.30	0.001
	2. Number of off-task glances M (SD)	13.95(5.97)	2.86 (1.55)	54.98	0.001
Comparison at Eight month corrected age	1. Duration of attention M (SD)	11.40 (9.90) **2.19 (0.65)**	33.31 (23.54) **3.32 (0.58)**	41.17	0.001
	2. Number of off-task glances M (SD)	13.95(5.97) **2.51 (.56)**	6.45 (3.10) **1.73 (0.54)**	35.83	0.001

Note. The values in bold are the means *M* and standard deviations *SD* of transformed data corresponding to the mean of the raw data.

Preterm infants were grouped on the basis of their medical risk, birthweights, and gestation age Resulting in two preterm infant groups (high risk and low risk for each of the risk factors). These groups were compared with each other and with the full term infant group. None of the full-term infants had high medical risk or were low birthweight.

The results of the ANOVA for the effect of birthweight on the performance of preterm infants on SA tasks are shown in table 4, table 5 and table 5 along with Tukey's HSD for the pair of groups.

No statistically significant differences were found between the low risk and high risk very preterm groups on any measures of SA. Both groups consistently obtained scores which were inferior to those of the full term infant group on all measures of SA. The differences between both high and low risk very preterm groups and the full term infant group reach statistical significance suggesting that prematurity per se may affect the aspects of SA development.

Preterm infants in all subgroups differed significantly from full-term infants on the two measures of SA, suggesting that even moderate levels of prematurity were associated with depressed performance on these measures.

Table 4. The Comparison of high risk, low risk infants and full-term infants on measures of sustained attention at eight months corrected age

Variables	High-risk preterm infants	Low-risk preterm infants	Full-term Infants	F	p	Tukey's HSD
(1) Duration of attention M (SD)	9.45 (4.30) **2.14 (.78) A1**	13.25 (13.08) **2.25 (.78)A2**	33.28 (23.44) **3.31 (.58) A3**	8.27	.00	A1 <. A3 (.00) A2 < A3 (.00)
(2) Off-task glances M (SD)	14.38(5.61)**B1**	13.52(6.40)**B2**	6.42 (3.10)**B3**	26.47	.00	B1 > B3 (.00) B2 > B3 (.00)

Table 5. The Comparison of extremely low birthweight, very low birthweight and full-term infants on measures of sustained attention at eight months corrected age

Variables	<1000 g birthweight (n=21)	1000-1500 g birthweight (n=16)	Full-term Infants (n=74)	F	p	Tukey's HSD
Duration of attention M (SD)	12.27(12.73) **2.24(.86) C1**	10.27 (4.08) **2.18 (.58) C2**	33.28 (23.44) **3.31 (.58)C3**	42.37	.00	C1 < C3 (.00) C2 < C3 (.00)
Off-task Glances M (SD)	14.66(6.72)**D1**	13.00(4.84)**D2**	6.42 (3.10)**D3**	37.93	.00	D1 > D3 (.00) D2 > D3 (.00)

Table 6. The Comparison of gestational age less than 28 weeks, 28-32 weeks gestations and full-term infants on measures of sustained attention at eight months corrected age

Variables	< 28 weeks M (SD) (n=15)	28-32 weeks M (SD) (n=22)	Full-term Infants M (SD) (n=74)	F	p	Tukey's HSD
Duration of attention M (SD)	11.11 (10.82) **2.24(.86) E1**	10.27 (4.08) **2.18 (.58)E2**	32.81 (23.31) **3.31 (.58)E3**	42.35	.00	E1 < E3 (.00) E2 < E3 (.00)
Off-task Glances M (SD)	14.54(5.97)**F1**	13.00(4.84)**F2**	6.45 (3.09) **F3**	40.42	.00	F1 > F3 (.00) F2 > F3 (.00)

Notes.
1. The values in bold are the mean *M* and standard deviation *SD* of transformed data corresponding to the mean and standard deviations of the raw data. Transformed data were used for the analysis due to the raw data were not normally distributed.
2. HSD: Tukey's Honestly Significant Difference Test. Only Tukey's HSD showing significant differences are reported.

Discussion

The present study found that preterm infants were inferior to full-term infants on SA tasks at both 10-11 month chronological age and eight month corrected age, but the differences in performance were much less when the infants were compared at the same corrected age. This suggests that maturation had a greater impact than exposure to environmental stimuli on the development of SA. However, as differences between the preterm and full term infants are statistically significant even when they were compared on corrected age. When PDI as a confounding factor was controlled for, the differences between very preterm and full-term infants on measures of SA remained.

Very premature birth seemed to adversely affect SA, those infants with higher perinatal risk factors such as a birthweight < 1000g or gestational age <28wks or serious medical complications performed no differently from larger more mature very preterm infants and those who had a relatively uncomplicated perinatal course. Given the small number of subjects these findings must be interpreted with caution. However to date this is the one of the few studies which has compared high risk and low risk preterm infants in terms of the development of a range of SA abilities in infancy. Previous studies have also reported that perinatal risk factors influence cognitive development however these have typically examined SA in older children and compared the development of children born preterm to that of children born full term (27).

Previous investigations of cognitive and general development have shown the importance of maturation in the development of preterm infants (28). Typically these studies, which focused on general development, language development and information processing, found that assessments made on the basis of corrected age showed no significant differences between the performance of preterm and full-term infants (29,30). The present study also found that preterm infants and full-term infants of the same corrected age did not differ in Bayley MDI scores and although a significant difference was found between preterm and full term infants on measures of SA these differences were far less than when assessment was on the basis of chronological age. These findings support the previous finding that maturation has a significant effect on the development of these abilities (31,32).

The present study found that preterm infants had deficits in SA at eight months corrected age. According to the theory of maturational lag (33), children who are at risk of subsequent learning difficulties and attention deficits may show delayed cognitive development during the first years of life. A number of studies reported that this developmental lag may manifest in young children in the form of delays in sensory-motor skills and visual-perceptual abilities (34). The present study found that preterm infants displayed significant deficits in the development of SA, which are core abilities underlying later cognitive development and learning.

In the current study, significant differences were found between preterm and full-term infants on measures of SA. Preterm and full-term infants also showed qualitatively different patterns of interaction with the objects presented to them.

Preterm infants were observed to have difficulty focusing their attention on the examination of the object as they spent shorter periods (duration of attention) of time in examining the objects than the full term infants. They also used less effective exploratory techniques compared to term infants and this is evident that they ceased the examination of the objects and averted their attention from the task more often than the term infants.

This pattern of behaviour may have important consequences. For example, Ruff (35) suggested that infants who explore less frequently and less effectively do not learn as much about the properties of objects and consequently will know less about them. Most studies have found these difficulties are more common in high-risk preterm infants than low-risk preterm infants at 14 weeks to 12 months (36,37). However in the present study, both low-risk and high-risk preterm infant groups (irrespective of the criteria used to determine risk status) differed significantly from full-term infants on attention measures. This conflicting finding could have been due to the fact that the low risk infants in the current study were at considerably higher risk than the low risk preterm infants in other studies (36,37).

Both low risk and high-risk preterm infant groups differed significantly from full-term infants on SA measures. This may be attributable to their early physical environment. In the NICU where most preterm infants spent the first 2-3 months of their lives, they were typically over-stimulated with high levels of light, sound and multiple painful procedures. They also experienced maternal separation for prolonged periods.

Gardner and Karmel (38) suggested that these adverse environmental conditions during the perinatal period may be associated with a lowered functional and structural coherence or integrity within the central nervous system and hence poor attentional skills. Experimental evidence from animal models has further shown that these adverse environmental factors in the perinatal period may lead to neuronal cell death in the immature brain (39). An EEG study on children who had attentional deficits found that these children showed excessively slow activity and decreased alpha power in the left and right hemisphere across the frontal, parietal, and temporal brain regions when they performed the Continuous Performance Task.

This suggests that they may have had a state of low central nervous system cortical arousal due to dysfunction in the subcortical centers (40). Volumetric measurement of brain regions in 8-years-old children born preterm showed disproportionately smaller volumes of the anterior cortical areas which are associated with increased incidence of attentional deficits and other behavioural disorders (41).

Subcortical brain regions appear to be involved in the regulation of the SA system (42). Biological and environmental insults associated with preterm birth may have resulted in differences in the architecture of these regions in preterm infants compared to typically developing full-term infants.

Conclusion

The findings of this study suggests that the deficits of sustained attention in preterm infants may be associated with birth prematurity per se, and that additional complications may not have any further detrimental effect.

References

[1]   Rickards AL, Kelly EA, Doyle LW, Callanan C. Cognition, academic progress, behavior and self-concept at 14 years of very low birth weight children. Dev Behav Pediatr 2001;22(1):11-8.

[2]   Van den Hout BM, Van der Linden D, Wittebol-Post D, Jennekens-Schinkel A, Van der Schouw YT, De Vries LS, et al. Visual, cognitive and neurodevelopmental outcome at 5 1/2 years in children with perinatal haemorrhagic-ischaemic brain lesions. Dev Med Child Neurol 1998;40:820-8.

[3]   Wolke D, Meyer R. Cognitive status, language attainment, and prereading skills of 6-year-old very preterm children and their peers: the Bavarian longitudinal study. Dev Med Child Neurol 1999;41:94-109.

[4]   Taylor HG, Klein N, Schatschneider C, Hack M. Predictors of early school age outcomes in very low birth weight children. Dev Behav Pediatr 1998;19(4):235-43.

[5]   Breslau N, Chilcoat H, DelDotto J, Andreski P, Brown G. Low birth weight and neurocognitive status at six years of age. Biol Psychiatry 1996;40:389-97.

[6]   Robson AL, Pederson DR. Predictors of individual differences in attention among low birth weight children. Dev Behav Pediatr 1997;18(1):13-21.

[7]   Ruff HA, Saltarelli LM. Exploratory play with objects: Basic cognitive processes and individual differences. New Dir Child Dev 1993;59:5-15.

[8]   Mirsky AF, Anthony BJ, Duncan CC, Ahearn MB, Kellam SG. Analysis of the elements of attention: A neuropsychological approach. Neuropsychol Rev 1991;2:109-45.

[9]   Barkley RA. Attention. In: Tramontana MG, Hooper SR, editors. Assess issues child neuropsychol. New York: Plenum Press, 1988: 145-76.

[10] Kelly TP. The clinical neuropsychology of attention in school-aged children. Child Neuropsychol 2000;6(1):24-36.

[11] Sergeant J. A theory of attention: An information processing perspective. In: Lyon GR, Krasnegor NA, editors. Attention, memory, and executive function. Baltimore: Paul H. Brookes, 1996:57-69.

[12] Mirsky. Disorders of attention: A neuropsychological perspective. In: Lyon GR, Krasnegor NA, editors. Attention, memory, and executive function. Baltimore: Paul H. Brookes, 1996:71-95.

[13] Aylward GP, Gordon M, Verhulst SJ. Relationships between continuous performance task scores and other cognitive measures: Causality or commonality. Assessment 1997;4:325-36.

[14] Swaab-Barnevele H, Sonneville LD, Cohen-Kettenis P, Gielen A, Buitelaar J, van Engeland H. Visual sustained attention in a child psychiatric population. J Am Acad Child Adolesc Psychiatry 2000;39(5):651-9.

[15] Ruff HA. Individual differences in sustained attention during infancy. In: Colombo J, Fagen JW, editors. Individual differences in infancy: Reliability, stability, prediction. Hilldale, NJ: Lawrence Erlbaum, 1990:247-70.

[16] Ruff HA, Saltarelli LM, Capozzoli M, Dubiner K. The differentiation of activity in infants' exploration of objects. Dev Psychol 1992;28(5):851-61.

[17] Ruff HA, Capozzoli M, Weissberg R. Age, individuality, and context as factors in sustained visual attention during the preschool years. Dev Psychol 1998;34(3): 454-64.

[18] Choudhury N, Gorman KS. The relationship between sustained attention and cognitive performance in 17-24-month old toddlers. Infant Child Dev 2000;9: 127-46.

[19] Ruff HA, Lawson KR, Parrinello R, Weissberg R. Long-term stability of individual differences in sustained attention in the early years. Child Dev 1990;61:60-75.

[20] Sun J, Mohay H, O'Callaghan M. Executive function in preterm and full-term infants. Early Hum Dev 2009;85(4):225-30.

[21] Ruff HA. Components of attention during infants' manipulative exploration. Child Dev 1986;57:105-14.

[22] Ruff HA, Lawson KR. Development of sustained, focused attention in young children during free play. Dev Psychol 1990;26(1):85-93.

[23] Noldus Information Technology. The Observer: System for collection and analysis of observational data. 3.0 ed. Wageningen, Netherlands: Noldus Information Technology, 1996.

[24] Bayley N. Bayley scale of infant development: Manual. 2nd ed. San Antonio, TX: The Psychological Corporation, 1993.

[25] Sanson A, Prior M, Garino E, Oberklaid F, Sewell J. The structure of infant temperament: Factor analysis of the revised infant temperament questionnaire. Infant Behav Dev 1987;10:97-104.

[26] Goldberg D. The general health questionnaire. Windsor, England: NFER-Nelson, 1981.

[27] Luciana M, Lindeke L, Georgieff M, Mills M, Nelson CA. Neurobehavioral evidence for working-memory deficits in school-aged children with histories of prematurity. Dev Med Child Neurol 1999;41:521-33.

[28] Hunt JV, Rhodes L. Mental development of preterm infants during the first year. Child Dev 1977;48:204-10.

[29] Bonin M, Pomerleau A, Malcuit G. A longitudinal study of visual attention and psychomotor development in preterm and full-term infants during the first six months of life. Infant Behav Dev 1998;21(1):103-18.

[30] Rose SA, Feldman JF, Wallace IF. Infant information processing in relation to six-year cognitive outcomes. Child Dev 1992;63:1126-41.

[31] Forslund M, Bjerre I. Growth and development in preterm infants during the first 18 months. Early Hum Dev 1985;10:201-16.

[32] Touwen BCL. The brain and development of function. Dev Rev 1998;18:504-26.

[33] Siegel LS. Infant tests as predictors of cognitive and language development at two years. Child Dev 1981;52:545-57.

[34] Fawer CL, Besnier S, Forcada M, Buclin T, Calame A. Influence of perinatal, developmental and environmental factors on cognitive abilities of preterm children without major impairments at 5 years. Early Hum Dev 1995;43:151-64.

[35] Ruff HA. Infants' manipulative exploration of objects: Effects of age and object characteristics. Dev Psychol 1984;20(1):9-20.

[36] Ruff HA, McCarton C, Kurtzberg D, Vaughan HG. Preterm infants' manipulative exploration of objects. Child Dev 1984;55:1166-73.

[37] Richards JE, Casey BJ. Development of sustained visual attention in the human infant. In: Campbell BA, Hayne H, Richardson R, editors. Attention and information processing in infants and adults. Hillsdale, NJ: Lawrence Erlbaum, 1992:30-60.

[38] Gardner JM, Karmel BZ. Attention and arousal in preterm and full-term neonates. In: Field T, Sostek A, eds. Infants born at risk. Boston: Allyn and Bacon, 1983: 69-98.

[39] Bhutta AT, Anand KJS. Abnormal cognition and behavior in preterm neonates linked to smaller brain volumes. Trends Neurosci 2001;24:129-32.

[40] El-Sayed E, Larsson J, Persson HE, Rydelius P. Altered cortical activity in children with attention-deficit/hyperactivity disorder during attentional load task. J Am Acad Child Adolesc Psychiatry 2002;41(7):811-9.

[41] Peterson BS, Vohr BR, Staib LH, Cannistraci D, Schneider KC, Katz KH, et al. Regional brain volume abnormalities and long term cognitive outcome in preterm infants. JAMA 2000;284:1939-47.

[42] Posner MI, Petersen SE. The attention system of the human brain. Annu Rev Neurosci 1990;13:25-42.

Chapter VI

Prefrontal lobe functioning and its relationship to working memory in preterm infants

Abstract

This chapter investigated working memory in preterm and full-term infants at 8 months after expected date of delivery. A case-control study design was used for the study. Thirty-seven preterm infants without identified disabilities and 74 full-term and gender matched healthy full-term infants participated in the study. All infants were assessed on working memory tasks at 8 months after the expected date of delivery (when preterm infants were actually 10-11 months chronological age). The findings of the study showed that preterm infants performed significantly more poorly than full-term infants at 8 months after the expected date of delivery on measures of working memory. The results suggest that the effects of maturation are greater than the effects of exposure to extrauterine environmental stimuli on the development of working memory. Furthermore, the preterm infants were divided into two subgroups on the basis of (a) low or high medical risk factors, (b) birthweight of < 1000 g versus 1000-1500 g, and (c) gestation age of < 28 weeks versus 28-32 weeks, in order to assess the effects of these variables on the performance of working memory. Medical risk, lower birthweight and lower gestation age were all found to adversely affect performance on working memory. The present study provides further insights into the emergence of working memory in infants and the feasibility of evaluating these abilities in infants who are at risk for further learning difficulties and attention deficits.

Introduction

Advances in medical technology continue to improve the survival rate of preterm infants, so that increasing numbers of children who weigh < 1000g at birth are surviving and entering the school system (1,2). These at-risk children have been the focus of much research and many follow-up studies have identified a strong relationship between birthweight and learning development at school age (3). Confounding this relationship, with the fact that as birthweight declines, the number and severity of perinatal complications experienced by infants is likely to increase, and the increased chance of having learning problems (4).

Extensive attempts have been made to identify sensitive predictors of later learning problems in both term and preterm children (5,6). It has been accepted that learning problems have multiple determinants, and it is important to consider the interactions of biological factors (such as medical complications and genetic endowment), environmental factors (such as demographic factors, quality of educational experience, socioeconomic, and psychosocial factors), and developmental factors (such as specific cognitive abilities and general development) (7). Frequently there is an association between perinatal risk and poor social circumstances. Several studies have demonstrated that social factors, particularly low educational level of the parents and socioeconomic status, play an important role in the intellectual outcome of both healthy full-term and preterm infants and those who had perinatal medical complications (8,9).

The population of Very Low Birthweight (VLBW, birthweight between 1001-1500 grams) and Extremely Low Birthweight (ELBW, birthweight less than 1000 grams or 750 grams) infants is known to be at increased risk for a broad spectrum of health and developmental problems, and also an increased incidence of psychosocial disadvantages (e.g., poverty, single parenthood, youthful maternal age, and limited parental education), producing a "doubly vulnerable" population, which places their development in even greater jeopardy (10). The assessment of subtle developmental and behavioural delays in infants is complicated, and currently there are few sensitive measures available for the early identification of learning problems in infants. Conventional developmental assessment tools, such as the Bayley Scales of Infant Development, (11) only provide global indicators of development and fail to measure specific skills that may provide sensitive predictions of later learning.

The assessment of specific cognitive skills, in particular working memory, rather than a global development score in infancy, has been advocated by a number of investigators (12,13). Working memory is defined as "the ability to maintain an appropriate problem solving set for the attainment of a future goal" (1). Working memory deficits have been linked to a range of developmental problems, including attentional deficit disorder (ADD), learning difficulties, and autism, all of which are more prevalent in children born preterm (14). Studying a group of infants at high-risk for learning difficulties should make it easier to identify factors that are predictive of later learning problems. This may lead to a greater understanding of the etiology of these problems in all children.

In Welsh and Pennington's model of working memory, certain information remains at the forefront of cognition, despite distraction, and hence is active for the purpose of guiding appropriate responses. An important characteristic of working memory is that it is prospective, that is, its purpose is to attain a goal. Fuster (15) suggested that this is achieved not only by holding information in mind, but also by guiding goal directed actions. Graham and Harris (16) stated that working memory is also necessary in tasks which require strategy selection, monitoring, and revision of actions. This implies that working memory not only enables information to be held in mind but also to be manipulated. It is generally agreed that these behaviours are governed by the prefrontal cortex of the brain (17). This part of the brain is late in developing and therefore may be particularly vulnerable to damage in preterm infants.

The development of frontal lobe in human infants

The prefrontal cortex is one of the last regions of the central nervous system to undergo full myelination, and developmental changes originating from frontal lobe development are evident in several periods of life (20). The most active periods of development of the prefrontal cortex appear to be in the first 2 years of life, then between 7 and 9 years, and finally in adolescence. The development of the frontal lobe in infants deserves particular mention because during this period remarkable and rapid changes occur in both the neural physiology and the behaviour of the human being. For the frontal cortex, the period of maximum synaptic excess appears to be in the second half of the first year (21), after which there occurs a protracted period of decline in synaptic density through selective elimination of little used pathways. Recent studies of human brain activity using Positron Emission Tomography (PET) documented developmental changes in rates of glucose metabolism (22). These changes are characterised by a rise in metabolism in the frontal region at approximately 6-8 months of age, followed by a prolonged period of decline in rates of metabolism which parallels the decline in synaptic density (22). Thus, it seems that the significant and rapid changes related to anatomy and function of the fontal lobe occur in the second half of the first year after birth and continue more slowly after this early period.

There is ample evidence that working memory also develops dramatically during the second half of the first year of life. For example, infants can hold information in mind for increasing periods of time and use this information to direct and regulate their responses. Behaviours of this type have been shown in numerous studies to be related to the prefrontal cortex.

Bell and Fox (23) further demonstrated a relationship between working memory and prefrontal lobe functioning and showed individual differences in frontal-brain electrical activity, as shown in EEG recordings and performance on the AB task which measures workingmemory. Infants at eight months of age who succeeded on the AB task exhibited greater power values in the frontal EEG during baseline recordings than infants who were unable to do the task (24).

Additional evidence for the importance of prefrontal cortex maturation for the development of working memory abilities has come from studies of children with phenylketonuria (25). Even when treated, this genetically transmitted error of metabolism can have the specific consequence of reducing the levels of the neurotransmitter dopamine in the dorsolateral prefrontal cortex. This results in impaired performance on tasks thought to measure working memory, such as the AB task (26). The standard AB task was originally described by Piaget (27) to measure the changes in the concept of object permanence in human infants. In Piaget's AB task, an infant sits before two identical hiding places, often referred to as occluders (e.g., two identical cloth covers or two identical lids) that are separated by a small distance. While the infant watches, a desired object is hidden in one location (A). After a delay, the infant is allowed to reach and search for the object. This hiding and search at location A is repeated. Then while the infant watches, the object is hidden at the second location (B). After the delay, the infant is allowed to reach and search for the object. Infants frequently make the error of searching again at location A, committing what is known as the classic AB error. Thus both electrophysiological and behavioural data provide support for the relation between the development of the prefrontal cortex and the emergence of working memory in the first year of life.

During this important maturation process, any damage or disturbance to the development of the prefrontal cortex due to disease, trauma, or conditions associated with perinatal risk factors (i.e., medical complications, extremely low birthweight, shorter gestation age) may lead to working memory dysfunction. Diamond and Goldman-Rakic (28) used animal models to examine whether lesions of the dorsolateral prefrontal cortex would have the same effect on infant monkeys as on adult monkeys. Two of the infant rhesus monkeys were tested longitudinally on the AB and the DR tasks. They received bilateral lesions of the dorsolateral prefrontal cortex at 5½ months. They were then tested on the AB task at 6 months. The findings showed that the infant monkeys that had the prefrontal lesions displayed poorer performance on the AB task than their age mates who did not have the prefrontal lesions. The lesions produced the same effect in infant monkeys as they did in adult monkeys with prefrontal lesions: they all reached incorrectly when the delay increased to 2-5 seconds s after the toy changed to the new hiding position.

Damage to the prefrontal lobe due to trauma and disease in infancy may have lifelong effects on working memory abilities, and may cause learning difficulties during school years (29). In comparison with adults, childhood frontal lobe lesions produce a more pervasive impairment, interfering with the acquisition of age-appropriate working memory skills. Most studies on the relationship between working memory development and frontal lobe damage in children are based on older children (30). However, a recent case study by Anderson, Damasio, Tranel, and Damasio (31) reported that an infant who had right frontal region damage at 3 months showed severe learning difficulties and behavioural problems at school, and failure in career development in adulthood despite average intelligence (as measured by traditional intelligence tests at school age and during adulthood). The study found that the impairments largely reflected a failure to develop working memory. These findings are consistent with the notion that early damage to prefrontal regions can lead to severe disruption of working memory, while not significantly affecting many aspects tapped by standard intelligence tests. They also suggest that the prefrontal cortex may have limited neuronal plasticity which contributes to poor working memory if the damage occurs early. This may be due to disruption to the laying down of the neural architectures which are viewed as the foundation of cognitive development. A detailed examination of the relationship between prefrontal cortex development and the development of working memory in a large sample of human infants has not been possible because of the relative lack of obvious prefrontal lesions in infants and the expense and lack of availability of neural imaging technology.

The prefrontal cortex of infants who are born preterm is even more immature and prone to damage from the multitude of adverse medical complications to which these frail infants may be exposed. Lesions or atypical development of the prefrontal cortex occurring as a consequence of these hazardous events may have a detrimental effect on the development of working memory which may have long-term consequences in terms of learning difficulties at school age. Indeed it has been found that children born preterm are at an increased risk for learning difficulties and attentional deficits when they reach school age and it has been suggested that this may be due to early abnormality in the development of the prefrontal cortex and consequently of working memory (32,33).

Failure of working memory has therefore been shown to underlie learning difficulties and attention deficits in children and these problems are particularly common in children born preterm. Historically, the assessment of working memory in infants was thought impossible. However, recent neuropsychological research has suggested that the AB task provide avenues for research on working memory.

This study was undertaken to compare the performance of preterm and full-term infants of the same corrected age (8 months) age and 10-11 month chronological age on tests related to working memory. Specifically the study tested two hypotheses:

- *Hypothesis 1:* There will be significant difference between preterm and full-term infants of the same chronological age in the performance of working memory task (i.e., exposure to extrauterine environmental stimuli is the key factor influencing the development of working memory.
- *Hypothesis 2:* There will be significant difference between preterm and full-term infants of the same corrected age in the performance of working memory task (i.e., maturation of the central nervous system from the time of conception is the key factors influencing the development of working memory).

Our research

This research involves the comparison of a cohort of ELBW infants (n = 37) and two comparison groups of full-term infants (n = 37 in each group) matched for gender and the age since expected date of delivery. The purpose of having two full-term comparison groups is to increase the statistical power. All infants were assessed on the working memory task. This measure formed the dependent variable. Infants were also assessed on the confounding factors that include the following perinatal variables: medical complications, birthweight, and gestation age. All infants were assessed on the above variables at 8 months after the expected date of delivery (preterm infants were 10 to 11 months chronological age at this time). Term infants were reassessed at an age equivalent to the chronological age of the matched preterm infants at the time of the first assessment. This retest provided a comparison with the preterm infants on the basis of chronological age.

Participants consisted of two groups – preterm and fullterm infants:

1. Preterm infants: The mothers of 41 preterm infants, who attended the Growth and Development Unit at Mater Children's Hospital in Brisbane, Australia, responded to an invitation to participate in this study. These preterm infants were all born at the Mater Mothers' Hospital, Brisbane, Australia, between May 1998 and July 1999. Inclusion criteria for preterm infants were:

- < 1500 g birthweight,
- < 32 weeks of gestation,
- eight months of age after expected date of delivery,
- no evidence of severe visual, auditory or neurological impairment, or severe congenital anomalies,
- living in the Brisbane metropolitan area, and
- mother was English-speaking.

Of the 41 preterm infants, 37 were included in the study group. Two infants were excluded from the study due to severe intellectual and neurological problems and two other infants were excluded from the data analysis due to errors in the administration of some of the test items. There were two sets of twins and one set of triplets. A "high medical risk preterm infant" was further defined as an infant who had one or more of the following perinatal medical complications, previously identified as associated with poor outcomes. (40,41). These were: Home Oxygen Dependency, Cerebral

Ventricular Hemorrhage, Ventricular Dilatation, and Periventricular Hemorrhage-Intraventricular Hemorrhage.

2. Full-term Infants: Names and addresses of potential full-term comparison infants who were the same sex as the matched preterm infants, born at the Mater Mothers' Hospital on the same expected date of delivery, were obtained from medical records at the hospital. Parents were then contacted by a letter, and provided with an information sheet, and a follow-up telephone call. A total of 207 letters were sent, and of these 74 mothers of infants with birth weights of > 2500g were selected to match the corresponding preterm infants on a first-come basis. Inclusion criteria for full-term infants were:

- > 2500 grams birthweight,
- 38-42 weeks of gestation,
- same sex as matched preterm infant,
- born on the same expected date of delivery as the matched preterm infant,
- no evidence of perinatal complications or congenital abnormalities,
- living in the Brisbane metropolitan area,
- mother was English speaking, and
- developmentally normal

In summary, all infants recruited into this study were born at the same hospital and tested at eight months (+ or - 2 weeks) after the expected date of delivery. Full term infants were reassessed when they were 10-11 month chronological age. All infants lived within a 50-kilometre radius of the Mater Mothers' Hospital and did not have identifiable disabilities at the time of assessment.

Participation in the project was voluntary and informed consent was obtained from at least one parent of each child. Ethical approval for the project was obtained from the Mater Children's and Mater Mothers' Hospital Ethics Committees, and the Queensland University of Technology Research Ethics Committee.

Working memory task

The assessment of working memory was based on a task derived from the AB and DR tasks which have been described in the literature (26, 34). In the AB task, an infant sits before two identical hiding locations (e.g., cloth covers, cups or wells) that are separated by a small distance. While the infant watches, a desired object is hidden in one location, location A. After a delay, the infant is allowed to reach and search for the object. This hiding and searching at location A is repeated. Then while the infant watches, the object is hidden at the second location, location B. After a delay, the infant is allowed to reach and search for the object. Infants frequently make the error of searching again at location A committing what is known as the classic AB error. The sequence of hiding locations in the DR task is random, whereas the hiding locations in the AB task are determined by the number of correct searches at location A. The administration procedure is described below.

1. *Materials.* The following materials were used for the Infant Working Memory task: one yellow cup (used to cover the toys), two red cups, three blue cups, and three small toys for hiding under the cups.
2. *Pre-test.* This involved the experimenter putting a toy on the table in front of the infant while the infant was watching. The infants were allowed to retrieve the toy immediately to test whether they could reach it. If it was unclear whether the infant had reached for the toy (e.g., if the infant showed an interest in the examiner or waited for several seconds before reaching to the toy), this procedure was repeated.

Ability to successfully retrieve the hidden objects is influenced by the infant's interest in and attention to the task (35). To maintain infant's attention to the task, the colours of the occluders (the cups under which the goal objects were hidden), were changed at set points in the test administration.

Administration of the infant working memory task

1-cup task. The Infant Working Memory task started with a 1-cup task. One yellow opaque cup and three small round toys were used. A toy was placed directly in front of the infant, at a distance of approximately 20 cm. While the child watched, the opaque yellow cup was placed by the examiner over the toy so that the toy was invisible.

For this trial and all subsequent trials the mother was asked to prevent the infant from reaching by gently holding him/her whilst the object was being covered and also during the imposition of a delay between hiding and retrieving the object. She was instructed, prior to the task, to release her child when the examiner said "find the toy." The infant's ability to remove the occluder and reach for the object underneath was then noted. Three trials were given for each of the delay periods (0, 4 and 10 seconds).

2-cup task. For the 2-cup task, two red opaque cups and the same three toys were used. One cup was positioned 11 cm to the right of the infant's midline, at a distance of 20 cm from the infant. The other was positioned 11 cm to the left, also at a distance of 20 cm from the infant. Testing began by positioning the goal object in front of the cup on the infant's left hand side. The cup was then moved to cover the object.

The infant was then permitted to retrieve the object and allowed a few seconds to play with it. The toy was hidden in the following positions: right, right, left, left, and right for the remaining 5 trials. Then the delay time between hiding the object and retrieving was increased to 2 seconds. For the 2 seconds delayed period trial, the order for hiding the toy was: right, left, left, right, right, and left. The hiding locations for the 4 s delay was the same as that of the 0 s delay and the hiding locations for the 10 s delay was the same as for the 2 seconds delayed time condition.

3-cup task. In the 3-cup task, three blue cups and the same toys were used. In this condition, the toy was always hidden to the left and the right side of the infant and never in the middle. The order for the hiding location was the same as for the 2-cup condition. For the 2- and 3-cup difficulty level, the toy was always hidden on the left side first, because perseverative reaching has been demonstrated to be more common on an infant's right side (36).

For the 1-cup task, three trials were presented at each time delay of the task. From the 2-cup to 3-cup Infant Working Memory task, six trials were presented at each time delay of the task. Three round toys with three colours (red, yellow, and blue) were used as objects for hiding under the cups. These three toys were used for each trial each for the first three trials at each time delay level based on the colour sequence of red, yellow, and blue. The procedure for the presentation of toys were the same for the second three trials at each time delay level.

During the inter-trial (i.e., between infant's retrieval and the preparation of next trial) interval, the experimenter gave the hidden toy to the infant to play with for approximately 20 s while the next trial was prepared. The inter-trial interval was about 20 seconds. A summary of the tasks is presented in table 1.

Table 1. Infant working memory task

Tasks	Number of hiding places	Occluder (cup/s)	Delay time between hiding and reaching	Location of hidden object					
1 cup	1	Yellow cup	Level 1: 0 s delay						
			Level 2: 4 s delay						
			Level 3: 10 s delay						
2 cups	2	Red Cups	Level 1: 0 s delay	L	**R**	R	**L**	L	**R**
			Level 2: 2 s delay	R	**L**	L	**R**	R	**L**
			Level 3: 4 s delay	L	**R**	R	**L**	L	**R**
			Level 4: 10 s delay	R	**L**	L	**R**	R	**L**
3 cups	3	Blue cups	Level 1: 0 s delay	L	**R**	R	**L**	L	**R**
			Level 2: 2 s delay	R	**L**	L	**R**	R	**L**
			Level 3: 4 s delay	L	**R**	R	**L**	L	**R**
			Level 4: 10 s delay	R	**L**	L	**R**	R	**L**

Note. R in the table refers to the right side, L refers to the left side of the infant. The bold type refers to the change to a new hiding position that provided a measure of inhibition to a prepotent response.

Criteria used for termination and continuation of the task

Each infant was tested on the 1-cup, 2-cup, and 3-cup tasks. In each of these conditions, the infant started from the easiest level of time delay, 0 seconds. If the infant failed to reach to the appropriate occluder on three consecutive trials at any delay level, the next trial was administered with one extra cup and 0 s delay, otherwise testing continued at the next level of delay with the same number of cups. The criteria used for terminating the task or moving to the next level are described in more detail below.

1. *1-cup task.* Three presentations of this task could be given at each time delay (0, 4, 10 s). If the infant succeeded in removing the cup and obtaining the object underneath within the time limit on at least two of three presentations, then the task was administered at next level of time delay. If the infant failed to obtain the object on all three

trials at a given time delay, following completion of three trials at 10 s delay the examiner moved on to the 2-cup task with a 0 s time delay.

2. *2-cup task.* Six presentations of the 2-cup task were given at each delay time. There were four delay times (0, 2, 4, and 10 s), making a total of 24 trials. If the infant succeeded in reaching to the correct position on at least three consecutive trials on a given time delay, the next level of time delay was then presented. During the 2-cup task, if the infant failed to reach to the appropriate occluder on three consecutive trials at any delay level, testing of the 2-cup task was terminated, and the 3-cup task was administered with 0 s time delay.

3. *3-cup task.* The criterion to pass this task was the same as in the 2-cup task. In this condition, if the infant failed to retrieve the toy on three consecutive trials at any delay level, the tester stopped the testing.

Scoring scheme for working memory

As shown in table 2, finding a hidden object in the 1-cup task requires infants to remember the hidden object rather than a location, and to be able to reach the hidden object. These are the criteria for the infants to perform the Infant Working Memory task. Finding a hidden object in location A in the 2- and 3-cup tasks requires working memory for location. Increasing the delay time between hiding and retrieval increases the difficulty of the task for infants (37).

Therefore working memory was scored on the memory for location, and this was scored on the basis of the 2- and 3-cup tasks in location A. A score of one was awarded if the infant remembered the location of the toy on the first trial of both 2- and 3-cup tasks, and on subsequent trials when the hiding position was the same position as on the previous trial (i.e., all the A trials which are the ones not in bold type in table 2).

The task administration was organised so that this was always the 1st, 3rd and 5th trial at each time delay level. The total number of correct trials from all A trials attempted was then calculated. Possible scores ranged from 0-12 for both the 2- and 3-cup tasks (i.e., a possible overall total range of 0-24).

All data were analysed using the SPSS package version 17.0. Each preterm infant had two comparison term infants matched for gender and age. The comparison between the study group and comparison groups on working memory tasks at eight months corrected age and 10-11 months chronological age was analysed by multivariate analysis of variance to test hypothesis 1 and hypothesis 2.

Table 2. Comparison of preterm and full-term infants on working memory tasks at 10-11 month chronological age and eight months corrected age

Executive function	Preterm	Full-term group	F	p
1.Working memory *M (SD)* *Chronological age*	5.75 (3.11) **1.67 (.57) A1**	13.42(4.01) **2.50 (.40) A2**	21.78	.00
2. Working memory *M (SD)* *Corrected age*	5.75 (3.11) **A1**	9.40 (4.45) **A2**	11.82	.00

If there was a significant difference between preterm and full-term infants, the confounding variables which may explain this difference were examined. Perinatal variables which might confound the effects of prematurity, such as medical risks, birthweight, and gestation age, were also examined using ANOVA to compare the differences between the two preterm and one full-term infant groups.

What we found

The aim of this analysis was to compare the performance of preterm and full-term infants of the same chronological age (i.e., 10-11 months after expected date of delivery) and the same corrected age (i.e., eight months after expected date of delivery) on working memory task. Table 2 provides the results on the comparison of preterm and full-term infants on working memory tasks at 10-11 months chronological age and eight months corrected age.

The univariate ANOVAs showed that each of the components of working memory contributed significantly to the differences between groups for working memory measure. There was a significant difference between the preterm group and full-term infants group on the working memory task.

There were significant differences between preterm and full-term infants at 10-11 months chronological age in the performance of working memory. Preterm infants showed significantly poorer performance than the full-term infant groups on working memory. These results supported Hypothesis 1, which stated that there will be significant difference between preterm and full-term infants of the same chronological age in the performance of working memory task (i.e., exposure to extrauterine environmental stimuli is the key factor influencing the development of working memory

It was also found that there were significant differences between preterm and full-term infant groups at eight months corrected age on working memory. Specifically, preterm infants as a group had significantly poorer performances on working memory compared with the full-term infant groups at eight months corrected age. These results supported hypothesis 2, which stated that the performance of preterm infants is different to full-term infants of the same corrected age on measure of working memory.

The next part of this study examined performance of infants at 8 months corrected age, and aim to identify those factors which might contribute to the differences in performance on working memory task between preterm and term infants. It is possible that some factors associated with being preterm affected performance of working memory more than prematurity per se. These factors include medical complications, lower birthweight and shorter gestation age. Further analyses were conducted to assess the effect of perinatal variables which might have significantly affected preterm infants' performance on the working memory measures.

Preterm infants were firstly grouped on the basis of their severity of medical complication as follows. None of the full term infants had serious perinatal complications and they were combined to form one group.

1. high-risk preterm group (n = 18), group 1;
2. low-risk preterm group (n = 19), group 2; and,
3. no medical complications (term infants n = 74), group 3.

The results of high risk preterm infants, low-risk preterm infants and full term infants are shown in Table 3.

The preterm infants who had a high medical risk in the perinatal period performed worse than those who did not have these medical risk factors on working memory, although the differences in performance were not statistically significant.

The scores of both the preterm infant groups were lower than those of full-term infants on working memory measure. These differences reached statistical significance between both groups of preterm infants and full-term infants on working memory. The difference between preterm infants who had high medical risk and full-term infants was greater than that between low-risk infants and full-term infants on working memory, suggesting that medical risk influences the development of working memory.

Table 3. The comparison of preterm infants at high medical risk, low medical risk, and full-term infants on measures of executive function and sustained attention at eight months corrected age

Variables	High-risk preterm infants	Low-risk preterm infants	Full-term Infants	F	p	Tukey's HSD
Working memory *M (SD)*	4.61 (2.95) **A1**	6.84 (2.93) **A2**	9.36 (4.22) **A3**	12.34	.00	A1 vs. A3 (.00) A2 vs. A3 (.03)

Table 4. The comparison of < 1000 g birthweight infants, 1000-1500 g birthweight infants and full-term infants on working memory measure at eight months corrected age

Variables	< 1000 g birthweight	1000-1500 g birthweight	Full-term Infants	F	p	Tukey's HSD
Working memory *M (SD)*	5.23 (3.36)**A1**	6.43(2.70) **A2**	9.36 (4.22)**A3**	11.01	.00	A1 vs. A3 (.00) A2 vs. A3 (.02)

Preterm infants were grouped on the basis of their birthweights as follows. None of the full-term infants was low birthweight and they were combined to form one group:

1. < 1000 g birthweight (n = 21), group 1;
2. 1000-1500 g birthweight group (n = 16), group 2; and,
3. normal birthweight group (term infants, n = 74), group 3.

The results of infants with less than 1000g birthweight, infants with 1001-1500g birthweight and normal birthweight infants are shown in Table 4.

The preterm infants who had < 1000 g birthweight performed worse than those who had ≥ 1000 g birthweight on working memory although the differences in performance were not statistically significant. The scores of both groups of preterm infants were poorer than those of full-term infants on working memory. These differences were statistically significant between both groups of preterm infants and full-term infants on working memory. Thus the differences between the preterm infants who had < 1000 g birthweight and full-term infants appear greater than that between the infants with ≥ 1000 g birthweight and full-term infants on working memory, suggesting that ELBW may significantly influence the development of working memory.

Preterm infants were grouped on the basis of their gestation age. None of the full-term infants had low gestation age and they were combined to form one group.

1. 28 weeks gestation age (n = 15), group 1;
2. 28 to 32 weeks gestation age (n = 22), group 2; and
3. normal gestation age (full-term infants, n = 74), group 3.

Table 5 shows that scores were poorer for the infants < 28 weeks gestation than for the preterm infants with ? 28 weeks gestation on working memory, and the scores of both groups of preterm infants were poorer than those of full-term infants on working memory. These differences reached statistical significance between preterm infants and the group of full-term infants on working memory.

Table 5. The comparison of < 28 weeks gestation infants, 28-32 weeks gestation infants and full-term infants on working memory measure at eight months corrected age

Variables	< 28 weeks M (SD)	28-32 weeks M (SD)	Full-term Infants M (SD)	F	p	Tukey's HSD
Working memory M (SD)	5.53 (2.66) A1	5.90 (3.43) A2	9.36 (4.22)A3	10.54	.00	A1 vs. A3 (.00) A2 vs. A3 (.00)

Discussion

Preterm and full-term infants of the same chronological age and same corrected age were compared on measures of working memory in order to assess the differential effects of maturation (biological maturity) and length of exposure to extrauterine environmental stimuli on the development of these abilities. Although a number of studies suggest that global development seems to be largely the result of maturational influence (38), others have reported that "neural sculpting" occurs as the result of exposure to environmental influences (39). Currently little is known about the impact of the environment on the development of brain mechanisms that mediate specific cognitive abilities, such as working memory.

It was found that preterm infants were inferior to full-term infants on working memory tasks at both the same chronological age and the same corrected age, but the differences in performance were much less when the infants were compared at the same corrected age. This suggests that maturation had a greater impact than exposure to environmental stimuli on the development of working memory. However, as differences between the preterm and full term infants remained even when they were compared on corrected age, other factors must also have impact on the development of working memory in these infants. It was also found that high-risk perinatal complications, extremely low birthweight (<1000 g) and very low gestation age (< 28 weeks) were associated with poor performance on working memory task.

Preterm infants represent a heterogeneous population which varies with respect to gestation age, birthweight, adequacy of interuterine growth, and the diversity of medical complications to which they may have been exposed. All too often in the literature these differences have been ignored and data from preterm infants has been lumped together. It is however essential to consider the effect which these factors may have over and above the effects of prematurity per se.

The perinatal risk factors examined in the present study were high medical risk, extremely low birthweight, and shorter gestation age. VD did not occur in any of the infants in the present study so it was not used for the analysis. Eighteen infants fell into this "high medical risk" category, and the remaining 19 preterm infants were defined as "low medical risk."

ELBW was defined as birthweight < 1000 g. Preterm infants in the < 1000 g birthweight group did not differ from the preterm infants with ? 1000 g birthweight group with regards to medical risk status. Two gestation age groups comprised infants with gestation age < 28 weeks and preterm infants with ≥ 28 weeks gestation age. Infants with gestation age < 28 weeks were regarded as having shorter gestation age. Likewise, preterm infants born at < 28 weeks gestation were not significantly different to those with 28-32 weeks gestation in terms of medical risk status. There was therefore an opportunity to consider the effect of birthweight and gestation age independent of medical complications.

In each case, the high-risk group (i.e., the medical complications group, the <1000 g birthweight group, and the < 28 weeks gestation group) performed more poorly than their low risk counterparts (i.e., the low medical risk group, the > 1000 g birthweight group, and the > 28 weeks gestation group) on working memory measure although these differences did not reach statistical significance. The performance of both the high risk and low risk preterm groups on measure of working memory were also consistently poorer than that of the full-term group, and this reached levels of statistical significance more frequently for the high risk preterm groups than for the low risk groups. The results of the effects of perinatal factors on the performance of working memory are summarised in Table 6 below. These findings suggest that medical risk, lower birthweight, and lower gestation age adversely affect performance on working memory measure.

Table 6. Influence of perinatal risk factors on performance of working memory measure when compared to full-term infants

Variables	Medical risk		Birthweight		Gestation age	
	High risk	Low risk	< 1000 g	> 1000 g	< 28 weeks	> 28 weeks
	p	p	p	p	p	p
Working memory	.03*	.00***	.00***	.02*	.00***	.00***

Note.The figures in the table above are summarized from Table 4, 5 and 6.
Significant difference between preterm infant group and full-term infant group:
*$p < .05$, ** $p < .01$, *** $p < .001$.

The findings of this study are consistent with those of other researchers, who have reported that perinatal risk factors influence cognitive development during the first year of life (42). Similar deficits in working memory have also been reported in studies of school age children who were born preterm and who experienced high medical risk (43). For example, Luciana et al [33] found that preterm born children at 7 to 9 years of age who had high medical risk differed from full-term infants on working memory tasks, and Taylor et al (44) also suggested that medical risk may influence the long term developmental outcomes of preterm infants.

The results are also consistent with previous studies of children with extremely low birthweight, whether defined as birthweight < 1000 g (32) or < 750 g (43), which have reported lower scores on the performance of working memory tasks. However the children in these studies were older than the children in the present study. The effect of Small for Gestational Age (SGA) may also influence the performance of working memory in the preterm infants with < 1000 g birthweight group in the current study. For example, the poorer performance of the ELBW infants on working memory may have been due to the fact that there were eight SGA infants in the ELBW group. Several studies, such as that of McCarton et al (45) have reported that SGA preterm infants tend to perform more poorly than their AGA counterparts on general developmental assessment measures. In the current study, SGA preterm infants tended to show poorer scores on the working memory measure than AGA preterm infants, but these differences did not reach statistically significant differences as the number of SGA infants in the present study was too small. Evidence for direct central nervous system effects of intrauterine undernutrition is primarily based on animal studies. Laboratory studies in rats and guinea pigs that have experienced intrauterine growth retardation have shown decreased brain weight, and reduced amount of brain DNA, protein, and myelin lipids (46). While extrapolation from animal studies is questionable this does raise the possibility that SGA infants may experience cognitive impairments as the result of reduced brain growth.

This study appears to be the first to examine the effect of gestation age on the performance of working memory. The effects of gestation age on subsequent cognitive development has been the topic of considerable debate. Many studies have included a heterogeneous group of preterm infants with a wide range of gestation ages. The effects of gestation age on subsequent development have consequently often been confounded by a higher incidence of perinatal complications and poor psychomotor development in the infants of lower gestation age (47, 48). In this study, both preterm infants with < 28 weeks gestation and infants with 28-32 weeks gestation had lower scores than the full-term infants on working memory. The differences between both preterm groups and full-term infants reached statistical significance on measure of working memory. This suggests that a shorter gestation age is no more detrimental to performance in these areas than prematurity per se.

There is considerable evidence that tasks which require the holding of information in memory involve the dorsolateral prefrontal cortex (49,50). The deficits in working memory observed in the high perinatal risk groups may be associated with the adverse effects of these perinatal risk factors on the prefrontal cortex which is very immature and sensitive in the preterm infants (51). Mouradian, Als and Coster (52) suggested that deficits in working memory might be due to late maturing cortical organization, particularly of the prefrontal regions. Myelination of the brain has been demonstrated to occur in a systematic fashion starting at the end of the first trimester and continuing at least until the end of the second year (53). Between 23 and 32 weeks of gestation, structural differentiation of the central nervous system is at its most rapid (i.e., neuronal differentiation, glial cell growth, myelination, axonal and dendritic growth and synapse formation). The preterm infants in the present study were born between 24 to 32 weeks gestation just at this time of brain development. Most of these preterm infants were in the Neonatal Intensive-care Unit for up to three months after they were born. The environment in the Neonatal Intensive-care Unit may not be conducive to the development of the brain and the perinatal risk factors which occurred during this period may have further adversely affect brain development. The prefrontal cortex, which appears to play a central role in regulating working memory, is a late maturing area of the brain, and is consequently likely to be particularly vulnerable to damage in preterm infants (54). Those preterm infants with these detrimental perinatal events are at particular risk for the abnormal prefrontal cortex functioning, hence the deficits in working memory.

The deficits of working memory observed in preterm infants may have long term consequences in terms of learning difficulties at school age. During school years, children born preterm who experienced high perinatal risks (i.e., high medical risks, extremely low birthweight, shorter gestation age) during the perinatal period have been found to have higher rates of deficits in cognitive and neuropsychological abilities, mathematics achievement, and adaptive behaviours, as well as higher rates of special education placements as compared with their full-term counterparts (2,33,44,55). It is possible that this is due to early abnormality in the development of the prefrontal cortex and consequent working memory impairment. Anderson et al (31) suggested that this might possibly result in inability to ever acquire aspects of working memory.

In summary, there were significant differences between preterm and full-term infants' scores on working memory at both 10-11 month chorological age and eight month corrected age. Medical risk factors, extremely low birthweight, and shorter gestation age confounded the effects of prematurity for working memory.

There are several limitations of this study. First, due to the restricted timeframe, long-term outcomes cannot be assessed. Hence a link cannot be made between the deficits in working memory in preterm infants found in the present study and learning difficulties in school. Second, the examiner was not blind to the preterm/term status of the infants and this may have affected the administration and coding of the tests. Third, the relatively small sample of preterm infants who could be recruited within the time constraints for the present study restricted the range of statistical analyses that could be carried out and thus limited their power. Finally, the strict selection criteria chosen to yield a group of relatively healthy preterm infants may have biased the sample and made it unrepresentative of the general population of every preterm infant. For the above reasons the results should be interpreted with some caution.

Conclusion

Differences were found between preterm and full-term infants on measures of working memory at both the same corrected and same chronological age. Maturation was found to be an important factor influencing the development of working memory. However other factors associated with prematurity were also found to affect performance on working memory measure. The present research examined the factors which may significantly affect the differences between preterm and full-term infants. In particular, high medical risk, lower birthweight, and shorter gestation age all affected the differences between preterm and full-term infants on of working memory measure.

References

[1]   Welsh MC, Pennington BF. Assessing frontal lobe functioning in children: View from developmental psychology. Dev Neuropsychol 1988;4(3):199-230.

[2]   Hack M, Friedman H, Fanaroff AA. Outcomes of extremely low birth weight infants. Pediatrics 1996;98(5):931-7.

[3]   Rickards AL, Kelly EA, Doyle LW, Callanan C. Cognition, academic progress, behavior and self-concept at 14 years of very low birth weight children. Dev Behav Pediatrics 2001;22(1):11-8.

[4]   Klebanov PK, Brooks-Gunn J, McCormick MC. Classroom behavior of very low birth weight elementary school children. Pediatrics 1994;94(5):700-8.

[5]   Aylward GP. Update on early developmental neuropsychological assessment: The early neuropsychological optimality rating scales. In: Tramontana MG, Hooper SR, eds. Advances in child neuropsychology. New York: Springer, 1994:172-200.

[6]   Ross G, Lipper E, Auld PAM. Cognitive abilities and early precursors of learning disabilities in very-low-birthweight children with normal intelligence and normal neurological status. Int J Behav Dev 1996;19(3):563-80.

[7]   Laucht M, Esser G, Schmidt MH. Developmental outcome of infants born with
      biological and psychosocial risks. J Child Psychol Psychiatr Allied Disciplines
      1997;38(7):843-53.
[8]   Roberts E, Bornstein MH, Slater AM, Barrett J. Early cognitive development and
      parental education. Inf Child Dev 1999;8:49-62.
[9]   Thompson RJ, Gustafson KE, Oehler JM, Catlett AT, Brazy JE, Coldstein RF.
      Developmental outcome of very low birth weight infants at four years of age as a
      function of biological risk and psychosocial risk. J Dev Behav Pediatrics
      1997;18(2):91-6.
[10] Aylward GP. Infant and early childhood neuropsychology. New York: Plenum Press,
      1997.
[11] Bayley N. Bayley scale of infant development: Manual, 2nd ed. San Antonio, TX:
      Psychol Corp 1993.
[12] Aylward GP, Pfeiffer SI, Wright A, Verhulst SJ. Outcome studies of low birth weight
      infants published in the last decade: A meta-analysis. J Pediatr 1989;115:
      515-20.
[13] McCall RB. What process mediates predictions of childhood IQ from infant
      habituation and recognition memory? Speculations on the roles of inhibition and rate
      of information processing. Intelligence 1994;18:107-25.
[14] Gathercole SE, Pickering SJ. Working memory deficits in children with low
      achievements in the national curriculum at 7 years of age. Br J Educ Psychol
      2000;70:177-94.
[15] Fuster JM. The prefrontal cortex: Anatomy, physiology, and neuropsychology of the
      frontal lobe. New York: Lippincott-Raven, 1997.
[16] Graham S, Harris KR. Addressing problems in attention, memory, and executive
      functioning. In: Lyon GR, Krasnegor NA, eds. Attention, memory, and executive
      function. Baltimore, MD: Paul H Brookes 1996:349-65.
[17] Goldman-Rakic PS. Specification of higher cortical functions. In: Broman SH,
      Grafman J, eds. Atypical cognitive deficits in developmental disorders: Implication for
      brain function. Hillsdale, NJ: Lawrence Erlbaum, 1994:3-17.
[18] Stuss DT. Interference effects on memory functions in postleukotomy patients: An
      attentional perspective. In: Levin HS, Eisenberg HM, Benton AL, eds. Frontal lobe
      function and dysfunction. New York: Oxford Univ Press 1991:157-72.
[19] Petrides M. Frontal lobe and working memory: Evidence from investigations of the
      effects of cortical excisions in nonhuman primates. In: Boller F, Spinnler H, Hendler
      JA, eds. Handbook of neuropsychology. Amsterdam: Elsevier Sci, 1994:59-82.
[20] Thatcher RW. Maturation of the human frontal lobes: Physiological evidence for
      staging. Dev Neuropsychol. 1991;7(3):397-419.
[21] Huttenlocher PR. Synaptogenesis in human cerebral cortex. In: Dawson G, Fischer
      KW, eds. Human behavior and the developing brain. New York: Guilford, 1994:
      137-52.
[22] Chugani HT, Phelps ME. Imaging human brain development with positron emission
      tomography. J Nucl Med 1990;32:23-5.
[23] Bell MA, Fox NA. The relations between frontal brain electrical activity and cognitive
      development during infancy. Child Dev 1992;63:1142-63.

[24] Bell MA. Frontal lobe function during infancy: Implications for the development of cognition and attention. In: Richards JE, ed. Cognitive neuroscience of attention: A developmental perspective. Mahwah, NJ: Lawrence Erlbaum, 1998:287-316.

[25] Diamond A, Prevor MB, Callender G, Druin DP. Prefrontal cortex cognitive deficits in children treated early and continuously for PKU.

[26] Monogr Soc Res Child Dev 1997;62(4):1-205.

[27] Diamond A, Doar B. The performance of human infants on a measure of frontal cortex function, the delayed response task. Dev Psychobiol 1989;22(3):271-94.

[28] Piaget J. The construction of reality in the child. New York: Basic Books, 1954.

[29] Diamond A, Goldman-Rakic PS. Comparative development of human infants and infant rhesus monkeys of cognitive functions that depend on the prefrontal cortex. Neuropsychol Abstr 1986;12:274.

[30] Scheibel RS, Levin HS. Frontal lobe dysfunction following closed head injury in children: Findings from neuropsychology and brain imaging. In: Krasnegor NA, Lyon GR, Goldman-Rakic PS, eds. Development of the prefrontal cortex: Evolution, neurobiology, and behavior. Baltimore, MD: Paul H Brookes, 1997:241-63.

[31] Eslinger PJ, Biddle K, Pennington B, Page RB. Cognitive and behavioral development up to 4 years after early right frontal lobe lesion. Dev Neuropsychol 1999;15(2):157-91.

[32] Anderson SW, Damasio H, Tranel D, Damasio AR. Long-term sequelae of prefrontal cortex damage acquired in early childhood. Dev Neuropsychol 2000;18(3):281-90.

[33] Harvey JM, O'Callaghan MJ, Mohay H. Executive function of children with extremely low birthweight: A case control study. Dev Med Child Neurol 1999;41:292-7.

[34] Luciana M, Lindeke L, Georgieff M, Mills M, Nelson CA. Neurobehavioral evidence for working-memory deficits in school-aged children with histories of prematurity. Dev Med Child Neurol 1999;41:521-33.

[35] Diamond A. Development of the ability to use recall to guide action, as indicated by infants' performance on AB. Child Dev 1985;56:868-83.

[36] Horobin K, Acredolo L. The role of attentiveness, mobility history, and separation of hiding sites on Stage IV search behavior. J Exp Child Psychol 1986;41:114-27.

[37] Hofstadter M, Reznick JS. Response modality effects: Human infant delayed-response performance. Child Dev 1996;67:646-58.

[38] Diamond A. Neuropsychological insights into the meaning of object concept development. In: Johnson MH, ed. Brain development and cognition: A reader. Cambridge, MA: Blackwell, 1993:208-47.

[39] Rutter M. Developing minds: Challenge and continuity across the life span. London: Penguin, 1992.

[40] Dawson G, Frey K, Panagiotides H, Yamada E, Hessel D, Osterling J. Infants of depressed mothers exhibit atypical frontal electrical brain activity during interactions with mothers and with a familiar nondepressed adult. Child Dev 1999;70:1058-66.

[41] Cohen SE, Parmelee AH, Beckwith L, Sigman M. Cognitive development in preterm infants: Birth to 8 years. J Dev Behav Pediatr 1986;7(2):102-9.

[42] Landry SH, Denson SE, Swank PR. Effects of medical risk and socioeconomic status on the rate of change in cognitive and social development for low birth weight children. J Clin Exp Neuropsychol 1997;19(2):261-74.

[43] Ross G, Tesman J, Auld PM, Nass R. Effects of subependymal and mild intraventricular lesions on visual attention and memory in premature infants. Dev Psychol 1992;28(6):1067-74.

[44] Taylor HG, Klein N, Minich NM, Hack M. Middle-school-age outcomes in children with very low birthweight. Child Dev 2000;71:1495-511.

[45] Taylor HG, Klein N, Schatschneider C, Hack M. Predictors of early school age outcomes in very low birth weight children. J Dev Behav Pediatr 1998;19(4):235-43.

[46] McCarton CM, Wallace IF, Divon M, Vaughan HG. Cognitive and neurologic development of the premature, small for gestational age infant through age 6: Comparison by birth weight and gestational age. Pediatrics 1996;98(6):1167-78.

[47] Neville HE, Chase HP. Undernutrition and cerebella development. Exp Neurol 1971;33(3):485-97.

[48] Duffy FH, Als H, McAnulty GB. Behavioral and electrophysiological evidence for gestational age effects in healthy preterm and full-term infants studies two weeks after expected due date. Child Dev 1990;61:1271-86.

[49] The Victorian Infant Collaborative Study Group. Outcome at 2 years of children 23-27 weeks' gestation born in Victoria in 1991-1992. J Pediatr 1997;33:161-5.

[50] Diamond A, Kirkham N, Amso D. Conditions under which young children can hold two rules in mind and inhibit a prepotent response. Dev Psychol 2002;38(3):352-62.

[51] Roberts JRJ, Pennington BF. An interactive framework for examining prefrontal cognitive processes. Dev Neuropsychol 1996;12(1):105-26.

[52] Diamond A, Lee E. Inability of five-month-old infants to retrieve a contiguous object: A failure of conceptual understanding or of control of action? Child Dev 2000;71(6):1477-94.

[53] Mouradian LE, Als H, Coster WJ. Neurobehavioral functioning of healthy preterm infants of varying gestational ages. Dev Behav Pediatr 2000;21(6):408-16.

[54] Battin MR, Maalouf EF, Counsell SJ, Herlihy AH, Rutherford MA, Azzopardi D, et al. Magnetic resonance imaging of the brain in very preterm infants: Visualization of the germinal matrix, early myelination, and cortical folding. Pediatrics 1998;101(6):957-62.

[55] Gilles FH, Shankle W, Dooling EC. Myelinated tracts: Growth pattern. In: Gilles FH, Leviton AD, Dooking EC, eds. The developing human brain: Growth and epidemiologic neuropathology. Baltimore, MD: Williams Wilkins, 1983.

[56] Taylor HG, Anselmo M, Foreman AL, Schatschneider C, Angelopoulos J. Utility of kindergarten teacher judgments in identifying early learning problems. J Learn Disabil 2000;33(2):200-10.

Chapter VII

Conclusion

Three major conclusions can be drawn from this study. Differences were found between preterm and full-term infants on measures of executive function (EF) and sustained attention (SA) at both the same corrected and same chronological age.

Maturation was found to be an important factor influencing the development of EF and SA. However other factors associated with prematurity were also found to affect performance on measures of EF and SA.

The present research examined the factors which may significantly affect the differences between preterm and full-term infants. In particular, low PDI scores, high medical risk, lower birthweight, and shorter gestation age all affected the differences between preterm and full-term infants on measures of EF but not on measures of SA.

The present study also examined the relationship between the components of EF, and the relation between EF and SA and general development. The lack of correlation among the components of EF suggests that they may be discrete abilities and further studies on the assessment of EF should fully assess all three components of EF. SA correlated negatively with planning in full-term infants but not preterm infants, which suggests that SA is only related to some aspects of EF depending upon the task demand, and may be also a discrete cognitive process. Neither EF nor SA measures correlated with general development which suggests that they are both independent of general development.

In summary, the present study used a case-controlled design to compare the performance on EF and SA in preterm and full-term infants at both the same corrected age and chronological age. Thus the influence of maturation and length of exposure to extrauterine environment on the development of EF and SA could be examined. Differences between preterm and full-term infants on measures of EF and SA were less at 8 months corrected age than at 10-11 months chronological age, suggesting that maturation has an important influence on the development of EF and SA. The present study also examined the confounding factors which may influence the differences between preterm and full-term infants in the performance of EF and SA and found that low PDI scores, high risk medical complications, lower birthweight, and shorter gestation age affected the differences between preterm and full-term infants on EF measures but not on SA measures.

The components of EF did not correlate with each other and SA only correlated with planning for the full term infants. Neither EF nor SA measures correlated with general development. All of these findings have significant theoretical and practical implications for future research and clinical practice.

Implications for early intervention programs and education

The survival rates of VLBW and ELBW preterm infants have increased dramatically over the years. As a consequence, increasing numbers of preterm infants are entering schools and experiencing learning problems. There is an urgent need to develop assessment tools to identify children who will experience learning problems before they reach school age, and to develop intervention programs to decrease or prevent the long-term impact of these difficulties. The deficits of EF identified in preterm infants indicate a critical need for further research to improve understanding of the causes of the deficits and their neurological foundations, thus creating a pathway for possible prevention of these problems.

First, medical intervention is required to decrease the incidence of high medical risk factors, lower birthweight, and lower gestation age which may directly cause prefrontal cortex damage or alter the maturation process of the prefrontal cortex, leading to executive dysfunction.

Second, if deficits in EF and SA can be detected in infancy it should be possible to develop appropriate intervention programs to minimise their later effects on learning. Education programs with a content which focuses specifically on developing working memory, inhibition, planning, and sustained attention abilities may assist these children.

Chapter VIII

Acknowledgments

The authors wish to acknowledge the support of Australian International Postgradue Research Scholarship to the first author. The authors also wish to thank Mater Children and Mater Mother's Hospital in Brisbane, Australia,for their support to provide the first author opportutnities to access preterm and full-term infantsto complete the executive function and sustained attention assessments.

Chapter IX

About the editors

Jing Sun, PhD, is a senior lecturer of School of Public Health at Griffith University in Australia. She has bachelor, master degree in education psychology and PhD degree in Neuropsychology. Her research interests are in child and adolescent health, employee's mental health, mental health promotion, biostatistics and epidemiology, with a particular focus on the mental health, multilevel and statistical modelling development, primary prevention in chronic diseases in national and international context. She has published extensively in international journals in areas of mental health promotion, entrepreneurships, prefrontal lobe functioning in infants, smoking cessation program, community based singing and meditative program in relation to chronic disease prevention, and resilience based programs. Email: j.sun@griffith.edu.au

Nicholas Buys, BA(Hons), MSc, PhD, Professor Nicholas Buys is the Dean, Leaning and Teaching in Health Faculty at Griffith University, Australia. He has a bachelor (Honours) degree in psychology, and master and PhD degrees in human rehabilitation. His research interests range from human rehabilitation, mental health, mental health promotion, to population health. He has published widely in international journals in areas of disability and work, mental health promotion in Australian Aboriginal and Torres Strait Islander people, social inequality in disadvantaged population, social inclusion, entrepreneurship, risk health behavior, and primary prevention of chronic disease. E-mail: n.buys@griffith.edu.au

Joav Merrick, MD, MMedSci, DMSc, is professor of pediatrics, child health and human development affiliated with Kentucky Children's Hospital, University of Kentucky, Lexington, United States and the Division of Pediatrics, Hadassah Hebrew University Medical Center, Mt Scopus Campus, Jerusalem, Israel, the medical director of the Health Services, Division for Intellectual and Developmental Disabilities, Ministry of Social Affairs and Social Services, Jerusalem, the founder and director of the National Institute of Child Health and Human Development in Israel. Numerous publications in the field of pediatrics, child health and human development, rehabilitation, intellectual disability, disability, health, welfare, abuse, advocacy, quality of life and prevention. Received the Peter Sabroe Child Award for outstanding work on behalf of Danish Children in 1985 and the International LEGO-Prize ("The Children's Nobel Prize") for an extraordinary contribution towards improvement in child welfare and well-being in 1987. E-mail: jmerrick@zahav.net.il

Chapter X

About Griffith Health, Griffith University, Queensland, Australia

Griffith Health at Griffith University has first-rate education and research programs with leading award-winning teachers and researchers contributing to the development of healthier communities.

Griffith Health provides:

- Undergraduate programs
- Postgraduate programs
- Research programs
- Continuing education programs

Griffith Health's high quality, innovative education programs range from the foundation health sciences to professional and clinical disciplines.It's teaching programs are supported by our world-class health research centres. Griffith Health is one of Australia's largest health faculties with over 7000 full time students enjoying state-of-the-art learning facilities and the most up-to-date teaching programs.

Griffith Health is committed to achieving excellence in public health research and postgraduate research training, and to developing high quality undergraduate and postgraduate courses of relevance to a changing society and recognised by professional bodies and accreditation authorities.

In the public health area Griffith offers a distinctive socio-ecological approach that integrates public, environmental and occupational health concerns with policy and service management considerations.At both the undergraduate and postgraduate level Griffith offers degrees that provide the knowledge and skills to work in a wide range of public health professions. Integrating knowledge and practice from a range of fields such as environmental health, health promotion, health services management and nutrition and dietetics. These degrees focus on the systems and practices that shape the health of nations, communities and individuals and the environments in which they live, work and take their leisure. Issues that help determine quality of life are investigated, such as globalisation, technology, environmental degradation and population trends, lifestyle and nutrition, control of existing and emerging communicable diseases, industry pollution management, food and drug safety.

Contact

Griffith Health
E-mail: health@griffith.edu.au

Chapter XI

About the National Institute of Child Health and Human Development in Israel

The National Institute of Child Health and Human Development (NICHD) in Israel was established in 1998 as a virtual institute under the auspicies of the Medical Director, Ministry of Social Affairs and Social Services in order to function as the research arm for the Office of the Medical Director. In 1998 the National Council for Child Health and Pediatrics, Ministry of Health and in 1999 the Director General and Deputy Director General of the Ministry of Health endorsed the establishment of the NICHD.

Mission

The mission of a National Institute for Child Health and Human Development in Israel is to provide an academic focal point for the scholarly interdisciplinary study of child life, health, public health, welfare, disability, rehabilitation, intellectual disability and related aspects of human development. This mission includes research, teaching, clinical work, information and public service activities in the field of child health and human development.

Service and academic activities

Over the years many activities became focused in the south of Israel due to collaboration with various professionals at the Faculty of Health Sciences (FOHS) at the Ben Gurion University of the Negev (BGU). Since 2000 an affiliation with the Zusman Child Development Center at the Pediatric Division of Soroka University Medical Center has resulted in collaboration around the establishment of the Down Syndrome Clinic at that center. In 2002 a full course on "Disability" was established at the Recanati School for Allied Professions in the Community, FOHS, BGU and in 2005 collaboration was started with the Primary Care Unit of the faculty and disability became part of the master of public health course on "Children and society". In the academic year 2005-2006 a one semester course on "Aging with disability" was started as part of the master of science program in gerontology in our collaboration with the Center for Multidisciplinary Research in Aging. In 2010 collaborations with the Division of Pediatrics, Hadassah Medical Center, Hebrew University, Jerusalem, Israel.

Research activities

The affiliated staff has over the years published work from projects and research activities in this national and international collaboration. In the year 2000 the International Journal of Adolescent Medicine and Health and in 2005 the International Journal on Disability and Human development of De Gruyter Publishing House (Berlin and New York), in the year 2003 the TSW-Child Health and Human Development and in 2006 the TSW-Holistic Health and Medicine of the Scientific World Journal (New York and Kirkkonummi, Finland), all peer-reviewed international journals were affiliated with the National Institute of Child Health and Human Development. From 2008 also the International Journal of Child Health and Human Development (Nova Science, New York), the International Journal of Child and Adolescent Health (Nova Science) and the Journal of Pain Management (Nova Science) affiliated and from 2009 the International Public Health Journal (Nova Science) and Journal of Alternative Medicine Research (Nova Science).

National collaborations

Nationally the NICHD works in collaboration with the Faculty of Health Sciences, Ben Gurion University of the Negev; Department of Physical Therapy, Sackler School of Medicine, Tel Aviv University; Autism Center, Assaf HaRofeh Medical Center; National Rett and PKU Centers at Chaim Sheba Medical Center, Tel HaShomer; Department of Physiotherapy, Haifa University; Department of Education, Bar Ilan University, Ramat Gan, Faculty of Social Sciences and Health Sciences; College of Judea and Samaria in Ariel and in 2011 affiliation with Center for Pediatric Chronic Diseases and Center for Down Syndrome, Department of Pediatrics, Hadassah-Hebrew University Medical Center, Mount Scopus Campus, Jerusalem.

International collaborations

Internationally with the Department of Disability and Human Development, College of Applied Health Sciences, University of Illinois at Chicago; Strong Center for Developmental Disabilities, Golisano Children's Hospital at Strong, University of Rochester School of Medicine and Dentistry, New York; Centre on Intellectual Disabilities, University of Albany, New York; Centre for Chronic Disease Prevention and Control, Health Canada, Ottawa; Chandler Medical Center and Children's Hospital, Kentucky Children's Hospital, Section of Adolescent Medicine, University of Kentucky, Lexington; Chronic Disease Prevention and Control Research Center, Baylor College of Medicine, Houston, Texas; Division of Neuroscience, Department of Psychiatry, Columbia University, New York; Institute for the Study of Disadvantage and Disability, Atlanta; Center for Autism and Related Disorders, Department Psychiatry, Children's Hospital Boston, Boston; Department of Paediatrics, Child Health and Adolescent Medicine, Children's Hospital at Westmead, Westmead, Australia; International Centre for the Study of Occupational and Mental Health, Düsseldorf, Germany; Centre for Advanced Studies in Nursing, Department of General Practice and Primary Care, University of Aberdeen, Aberdeen, United Kingdom; Quality of Life Research Center, Copenhagen, Denmark; Nordic School of Public Health, Gottenburg, Sweden, Scandinavian Institute of Quality of Working Life, Oslo, Norway; Centre for Quality of Life of the Hong Kong Institute of Asia-Pacific Studies and School of Social Work, Chinese University, Hong Kong.

Targets

Our focus is on research, international collaborations, clinical work, teaching and policy in health, disability and human development and to establish the NICHD as a permanent institute at one of the residential care centers for persons with intellectual disability in Israel in order to conduct model research and together with the four university schools of public health/medicine in Israel establish a national master and doctoral program in disability and human development at the institute to secure the next generation of professionals working in this often non-prestigious/low-status field of work.

Contact

Joav Merrick, MD, DMSc
Professor of Pediatrics, Child Health and Human Development
Medical Director, Health Services,
Division for Intellectual and Developmental Disabilities,
Ministry of Social Affairs and Social Services,
POB 1260, IL-91012 Jerusalem, Israel.
E-mail: jmerrick@zahav.net.il

Chapter XII

About the book series "Pediatrics, child and adolescent health"

Pediatrics, child and adolescent health is a book series with publications from a multidisciplinary group of researchers, practitioners and clinicians for an international professional forum interested in the broad spectrum of pediatric medicine, child health, adolescent health and human development.

- Merrick J, ed. Child and adolescent health yearbook 2011. New York: Nova Science, 2012.
- Merrick J, ed. Child and adolescent health yearbook 2012. New York: Nova Science, 2012.
- Roach RR, Greydanus DE, Patel DR, Homnick DN, Merrick J, eds. Tropical pediatrics: A public health concern of international proportions. New York: Nova Science, 2012.
- Merrick J, ed. Child health and human development yearbook 2011. New York: Nova Science, 2012.
- Merrick J, ed. Child health and human development yearbook 2012. New York: Nova Science, 2012.
- Shek DTL, Sun RCF, Merrick J, eds. Developmental issues in Chinese adolescents. New York: Nova Science, 2012.
- Shek DTL, Sun RCF, Merrick J, eds. Positive youth development: Theory, research and application. New York: Nova Science, 2012.

- Zachor DA, Merrick J, eds. Understanding autism spectrum disorder: Current research aspects. New York: Nova Science, 2012.
- Ma HK, Shek DTL, Merrick J, eds. Positive youth development: A new school curriculum to tackle adolescent developmental issues. New York: Nova Science, 2012.
- Wood D, Reiss JG, Ferris ME, Edwards LR, Merrick J, eds. Transition from pediatric to adult medical care. New York: Nova Science, 2012.

Contact

Professor Joav Merrick, MD, MMedSci, DMSc
Medical Director, Medical Services
Division for Intellectual and Developmental Disabilities
Ministry of Social Affairs and Social Services
POBox 1260, IL-91012 Jerusalem, Israel
E-mail: jmerrick@zahav.net.il

Index

N

O

P